Dailey
Strengthening

"*Dailey Strengthening* has improved my posture, balance, standing, and walking, and it eased my challenge of living with MS. If you question whether an inner body workout can change your life, suspend your disbelief long enough to try it. Watch as miracles begin to happen. Change your mind, change your body, and ultimately, you will change your attitude and how you react to life. Thank you, Alice Ann! It is a must-read and a workout for anyone wanting wellness from the inside out."

—JACKIE WALDMAN

Author of *The Courage to Give* series

"On paper, I am an eighty-eight-year-old woman with severe scoliosis. After practicing *Dailey Strengthening* with Alice Ann, people now look at me and ask, 'What are you doing? You look so young! Your posture is amazing!' Today, I am an eighty-eight-year-young woman with energy and a zest for life. Alice Ann's work is life changing. Her methods for attaining correct posture and correct methods for standing and walking have increased my body awareness, my balance, and my overall well-being. I recommend her book to all wanting to experience, as Alice Ann says, 'mind over matter and matter minds!'"

—SARAH YARRIN

Student, Oasis Mind-Body Conditioning Center

"This amazing body of work has taken Alice Ann years to gather, experience, and teach. No matter what body type you are or what you want to change, you'll find your answers in *Dailey Strengthening*. It is a true blessing for all of us."

—ROBERTA REINECKE

Instructor of Physio-Synthesis

Dailey
Strengthening

6 Keys to Balance Core Muscles for Optimal Health

Alice Ann Dailey

with illustrations by Megan Dailey

BROWN BOOKS
PUBLISHING GROUP

Dailey Strengthening:
6 Keys to Balance Core Muscles for Optimal Health

Brown Books Publishing Group
16250 Knoll Trail Drive, Suite 205
Dallas, Texas 75248
www.BrownBooks.com
(972) 381-0009

A New Era in Publishing™

ISBN 978-1-61254-864-7
Library of Congress Control Number 2015948045

Printed in the United States
10 9 8 7 6 5 4 3 2 1

Illustrations by Megan Dailey, Graphic Designer

For more information or to contact the author, please go to www.DaileyStrengthening.com.

TABLE
OF CONTENTS

PART ONE: HEALTH AWARENESS

Ingredients for Good Health   **1**
Getting the Body in Shape   5
The Body's Regulatory Mechanism for Hunger & Thirst   8
Body Shape & Endocrine System Connection   12
Another Perspective on Body Types & Weight Gain   13
A Popular Habit Ayurveda Prohibits   16

Health Problems   **17**
Liver & Gallbladder Flush   17
Hearing Loss   19
Carpal Tunnel Syndrome & Vitamin B6   21
Macular Degeneration & Nutrition   22
Low Salt Intake & Health   23
Cortisone   25
Health Benefits from Nutritional Supplements   26
Side Effects of Medicines   27

Cancer & Oxygen   **29**
The Power of Posture   30
Respiration   39
The Influence of Mind over Matter   46
The Beginning of the Mind-Body Connection   46
The Importance of Healthy Feet   49
Corrective Change Discomfort   52
Healing for a Stressed Mind & Body   53

Too Much Exercise, Too Little Education   **56**

Overall Physical Fitness   62

Meditation 101   67

Kinesthetic Awareness   70

PART TWO: THE WAY IT WORKS

Dailey Inner Core Workout   **73**

Triangles   78

Inner Core Workout Structural Balance Training   **99**

Foot Movements   102

Leg Rotations   111

Hip Lift   117

Knee Spreads   118

Leg Spreads   124

Pelvic Tilts & Lifts   126

Head Lifts   130

Reversals of the Spine & Neck   133

Chin Lifts   135

Reversals   139

Cat Positions   142

Shoulder Movements   145

Arm Exercises   149

Arm Rotations   150

Circle Arm Movements   155

Forward & Backward Sways   163

Forward Bends   166

Rotational Movements   171

Lateral Bends   177

Knee Bends   180

PART THREE: LESSON PLANS

Dailey Inner Core Workout Lesson Plans	**185**
Plan 1	186
Plan 2	188
Plan 3	190
Plan 4	192
Plan 5	194
Plan 6	196
Plan 7	198
Plan 8	200
A Parting Word	**203**
References	**204**
Acknowledgments	**207**
About the Author	**209**
Index of Illustrations	**211**

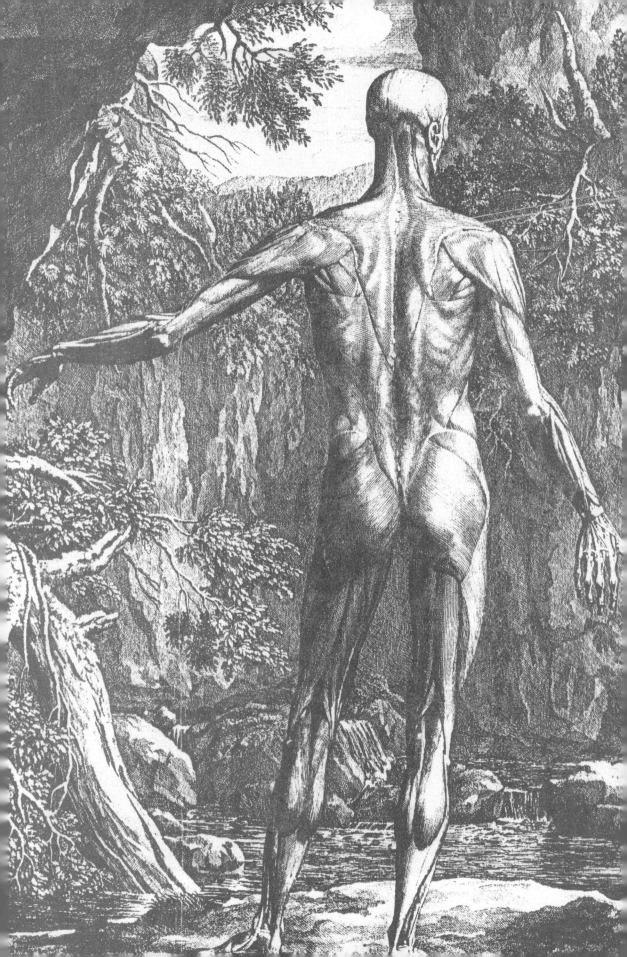

PART ONE
HEALTH
AWARENESS

"THE DOCTORS OF THE FUTURE WILL GIVE NO MEDICINE, BUT WILL
INTEREST HIS [SIC] PATIENTS IN THE CARE OF THE HUMAN FRAME,
IN DIET, IN THE CAUSE AND PREVENTION OF DISEASE."

—ATTRIBUTED TO
THOMAS ALVA EDISON

INGREDIENTS FOR GOOD HEALTH

John Naisbitt, in his book *Megatrends*, states that one of the major trends transforming American society is the shift in health care from institutional help to self-help. Health care providers often recommend medications and surgery for physical ailments. The most effective way people can take care of their own health and prevent future illness and pain is to practice proper joint positioning. We are seldom aware that our joints are misaligned due to habitual overstressing of muscles, which may cause many forms of discomfort and illness. All of our organs, glands, and systems (respiratory, nervous, immune, lymph, muscular, skeletal, endocrine, and cardiovascular) are affected by our body alignment. When such misalignment is habitual, we must re-learn proper joint positioning. If we don't invest time now in taking care of our bodies, we will eventually spend more time, money, and energy trying to fix the resulting health issues later. An ounce of prevention is worth a pound of cure.

The purpose of writing this book is to provide the knowledge that I have gained from my students and teaching experience to every person who wants to learn about a natural, healthy form of movement, as well as how to maintain the health of the human frame and body systems.

As the trend for self-help progresses, it becomes increasingly important to learn about the ingredients necessary for good health. It is essential for everyone to be physically active. Physical activity produces greater benefits based on *how* you move rather than *how much* you move. How you walk, stand, and sit can lead to wellness or illness. To make a change toward wellness and disease prevention, you must learn the difference between balanced and unbalanced alignment when walking, standing, and sitting. These preventive procedures are mostly limited to costly medical tests for early diagnoses of cancer, disease, and other physical problems. Learning how to prevent health problems by regularly performing the right exercise program is requisite to making a change toward wellness and disease prevention.

In my years of practice since 1985, when I graduated with an MS in exercise physiology and a minor in nutrition, I have witnessed many physical success stories, including recovery from motion sickness, migraine headaches, urinary incontinence, stress, weight gain, back/knee/shoulder/hip pain, and more. Recovery was achieved by the implementation of core muscle strengthening, posture correction, structural support, flexibility, and body-awareness training. I personally have experienced joint pain in six areas of my body at different times over the years; however, now that I am officially at retirement age, I have no pain in any area. The neuromuscular reeducation technique that solved the problems was my Dailey Inner Core Workout, based on a method created in the 1930s by Amy Cochran, an MD trained in osteopathy who noticed that many of her patients had poor posture and lack of muscle tone. The *key* to her method was based on *six triangles* of body alignment.

The Dailey Inner Core Workout is a revision of her method that helps people improve communication between the mind and body, as well as understand what is causing their discomfort and how to solve their problem. It is the only self-help method of its kind in the US, and it is successful for people of all ages and fitness levels. The movements reconstruct a misaligned body into balanced postural alignment.

Our lifestyle has changed since the early 1900s. Many of our six-hundred-plus muscles have been underused or unemployed. We must get all of our muscles back to work; however, good health is more than possessing an active, strong, flexible, and balanced body. We must gather information that is essential for us to make healthy choices. The earlier in life we start making healthy choices, the more likely we will be to continue to have a low risk for illness and disease. Medical research changes so quickly that often what was believed to be true five to ten years ago can be easily refuted today. When I worked as an office assistant at the University of Texas Southwestern Medical Center at Dallas, a research scientist told me, "Science is like an umpire. They call it as they see it, and that is what it becomes."

There is a profusion of information available about fitness in books, magazines, newspapers, and television. If we are to become more responsible for our health, we must also be responsible for sifting through the plethora of fitness information to make intelligent decisions about which changes will ultimately benefit our quality, as well as our longevity, of life. This abundance of information comes from many sources—some more qualified than others. Who are some of these people who are prescribing exercise and nutrition to the masses? What are their qualifications, and what is the basis and substance of their prescriptions? Do they actually possess the knowledge and professional working experience of dealing with many types of people who exhibit various levels of physical conditioning?

An important issue to consider—which has had very little notice from the media to date—concerns the balance of three components of physical conditioning: cardiovascular endurance, weight training, and flexibility.

> *Cardiovascular endurance* and aerobic exercise have been publicized extensively. Today, more people are running, walking, aerobic dancing, and swimming. Participants in these activities are making strong inroads in the prevention of cardiovascular disease.

> *Strength* is another component of physical fitness, and, in recent years, weight training has become more popular.

> *Flexibility*, the third component of physical conditioning, is equally as necessary as cardiovascular endurance and strength (which all become increasingly important with age).

Cardiovascular endurance, strength, and flexibility each play important roles in conditioning, and all three should be incorporated into a well-balanced exercise program. The same reasoning that requires carbohydrates, proteins, and fats to be balanced in our diet can also be applied to physical conditioning—an excess or deficit in any element results in its own special problem. Flexibility, along with correct body mechanics, must be balanced with aerobic- and strength-training activities. This type of exercise program produces a synergistic effect, making each component much stronger than it would be if one of the elements was neglected.

Another reason for incorporating flexibility and proper biomechanics principles into your exercise program is to maintain a healthy back. Through years of poor posture (incorrect body mechanics), many people develop muscular imbalance and joint compression, resulting in lower back pain. Fortunately, this condition can be prevented.

Most people experience back pain before they realize the importance of flexibility and good body mechanics—training by crisis rather than prevention. An alarming 80 percent of the adult population eventually experiences back pain. It secondarily affects cardiovascular disease and aerobic activities through the incapacitation of injured runners, frequently caused by poor biomechanics in their running stride. Strength training is also compromised by a weak back.

To keep your body sound and free from injury or pain, consider putting balance into your exercise program. It's up to you.

Getting the Body in Shape

If each person were reduced to his or her skeletal structure, we would all look fairly alike. The long bones would vary in length and circumference. The shoulder and pelvic girdles would vary in width, but generally, the skeletal structures would be very similar.

Even in young children, there is not much variance in body shapes, excluding the basic ectomorphic and mesomorphic classification of body types that measures the degree of muscularity and bone development. Muscle, connective tissue, and adipose (fat) tissue, as well as skeletal structure, are organized to give each person a unique shape. No matter what degree of slenderness or muscularity, the bodies of healthy, young children are sleek and toned. Each form is well designed. So what happens to these well-organized structures we begin with? We don't know enough about them and how to maintain them.

Philosopher Arthur Schopenhauer said, "To neglect one's body for any other advantage in life is the greatest of follies."

The degenerating process is so gradual that before we are conscious of what is happening, we may try on a pair of last season's slacks and find that the waistband is too tight. Our body has become flabby and overweight. Then we frantically run to the "hardest" exercise class we can find to sweat off the unwanted fat. This method seldom works for several reasons.

In a study conducted at the Institute for Aerobics Research at Cooper Center in Dallas by R. Donald Hagan, et al., it was found that after a twelve-week period, the body fat of exercising and control groups of men and women remained constant, while the dieting groups' body fat decreased 4.0 percent for men and 4.6 percent for women. The dieting and exercising group had a decrease of 5.9 percent for men and 5.2 percent for women.

Another factor in the reduction of body fat through exercise is that fat is not the only source of fuel used by the body for energy. The major energy-supplying nutrient is from carbohydrates, which are converted in the body to glycogen and glucose. The next sources are from fats converted to fatty acids and, as a last resort, proteins, which are converted to amino acids.

The fuel used for a specific type of exercise is dependent to some extent on what type of skeletal muscle fiber is involved in the exercise. Fast twitch muscle fibers—which are adapted to short, explosive bursts of contractions such as jumps; weight training; sprints in track, field, and swimming; as well as rapid movements in team sports—tend to rely on creatine phosphate stored in the muscle and the anaerobic breakdown of muscle glycogen and blood glucose. Slow twitch fibers, unlike extreme muscle contractions in weight training, are used more in less extreme contractions for endurance events such as running, swimming, rowing, cycling, and most of the running action in basketball, football, and soccer—team sports that require repetitive contractions over a long period of time. These endurance activities are more apt to burn fat, glycogen, and glucose aerobically.

According to the book *Physiology of Exercise*, if a person performs heavy exercise—for example, in an aerobic exercise class for 40 to 120 minutes—only one-fourth of the calorie expenditure is from fatty acids. The remaining energy is supplied by the aerobic breakdown of muscle glycogen and blood glucose. As hard work is prolonged—for example, more than 120 minutes, as in a marathon race—a greater contribution of the fuel comes from fat stored in muscle cells and from fatty acids in the blood. This increased use of fat is a gradual process but may account for 25 percent of the energy demands after one hour of exhaustive work and more than 50 percent after four hours.

Remember, with light exercise, slow twitch fibers are activated more than fast twitch fibers, so nearly all of the energy is released by the aerobic breakdown of fat, glycogen, and glucose. As the duration of light exercise increases, so does the role played by the combustion of free fatty acids for energy. For example, one who walks continuously for eight hours may supply up to 90 percent of his energy needs by the aerobic breakdown of fatty acids at the end of eight hours but only 25 to 50 percent during the first four hours of work. This suggests that as exercise is prolonged, an increasing recruitment of slow twitch fibers and an increasing activation of enzymes are involved in fatty acid breakdown.

Another reason exercise may not be the only process of getting back into shape is that we're approaching "getting fit" from the wrong angle. If the primary focus were on health, it would take care of getting "in shape." A shapely, youthful body will come automatically when you have a healthy lifestyle. A healthy body is not overweight or out of shape. It is important to quit thinking about weight and begin thinking about health.

The Body's Regulatory Mechanism for Hunger & Thirst

You may be tired of hearing about nutrition from the media, but it is the next consideration of getting healthy. Most of our food is so processed and refined, grown with chemical fertilizers on nutrient-deficient soils, sprayed with pesticides, and applied with dyes and preservatives that the food value we are getting is insufficient to supply our bodies with the nutrients we need to maintain health. We have become malnourished. In the short term, we can't do much about the fertilizers, pesticides, and poor soil, but we can do something about processed food—do not buy it! Shop around the edges of the grocery store for fresh or frozen foods, vegetables, and fruits, not down the aisles where most of the packaged, processed foods are found.

We have gotten our blood sugar and glandular (endocrine) system so out of balance that we crave all kinds of foods we think we can't live without. If you crave a particular kind of food, you are not getting the nutrients needed to create a feeling of satiety, or fullness to the point of satisfaction. Let's explore the mechanism by which we experience hunger, acquire an appetite, or develop preferences for certain types of foods and reach a sense of satiety after eating.

There are three areas in the brain that regulate the intake of food and liquids—the hunger center, the satiety center, and the thirst center. They are all located in the hypothalamus. We become hungry when our blood sugar decreases to a critical level. We have an appetite for a certain food when the nutrient level the desired food supplies decreases to a critical level.

Thirst is less complex than hunger. When our bodies become dehydrated, we feel the sensation of thirst. That is when the fluid of the body decreases to a critical point in proportion to the increase of solids and sodium in the fluid. The concentration is monitored by the thirst center, which at a critical level produces an electrical stimulation causing a person to consciously experience thirst and take the steps necessary to accomplish the act of drinking.

You receive relief from thirst immediately after drinking water, even before the water has been absorbed from your gastrointestinal tract. How does this happen? After you ingest water, it may take thirty minutes to an hour for all the water to be absorbed and distributed throughout your body. Therefore, a system for temporary relief of thirst is necessary to ensure you will not continue to drink more and more. The partial relief of thirst, lasting about fifteen minutes, is caused by the act of drinking. Distension of your stomach and other portions of the upper gastrointestinal tract provide additional temporary relief from thirst. For instance, studies have shown that the simple inflation of a balloon in the stomach can relieve thirst for five to thirty minutes. Without this short-term relief system, a person would continue to drink. With the long-term and short-term systems of relieving thirst, a person can become accurately rehydrated.

It is well known that a thirsty animal almost never drinks more than the amount of water needed to relieve the state of dehydration. Man has the same regulatory mechanism. A person continually becomes dehydrated, causing the volume of extracellular (outside the cells) fluid to decrease and its concentration of sodium and other elements to rise. When the sodium concentration rises to a certain level above normal, the thirst center is tripped, producing a level of thirst strong enough to activate the necessary motor effort to cause drinking. The person ordinarily drinks precisely the required amount of fluid to bring the extracellular fluids back to normal—that is, to a state of satiety.

The body's hunger-appetite-satiety centers regulate nutrition just as the thirst center regulates fluid, although nutritional regulation is much more complicated than fluid regulation due to the many different nutrients being monitored. When nutrient stores of the body fall below normal, the hunger center in the hypothalamus becomes highly active and the person experiences increased hunger. Conversely, when the nutrient stores are abundant, the person loses hunger and develops a state of satiety.

One of the nutritional factors that controls the degree of activity of the hunger center is the availability of glucose to body cells. A decrease in blood glucose or blood sugar concentration is associated with the development of hunger. Observations have shown that an increase in blood sugar increases measured electrical activity in the satiety center while it decreases electrical activity in the hunger center. In other words, an increase in blood sugar increases a feeling of fullness and decreases hunger. In the same manner, an increase in amino acid and protein concentration in the blood reduces hunger, as do free fatty acids.

Nutritional regulation also involves long-term and immediate short-term systems. In short-term regulation, when a reasonable quantity of food has passed through the mouth, the degree of hunger is decreased. It is postulated that various brain factors relating to feeding, such as chewing, salivation, swallowing, and tasting, "meter" the food as it passes through the mouth. After a certain amount has passed through, the brain's hunger center becomes inhibited, usually lasting twenty to forty minutes. Gastrointestinal filling, or a full stomach, also inhibits the hunger center and is more intense and longer-lasting than the head factors.

Long-term regulation of food intake is concerned with maintenance of normal quantities of nutrient stores in body tissues. Vitamins A, D, E, and K are soluble in fats and are stored in various tissues, including the liver. Water-soluble vitamins—the vitamin B group and vitamin C—are not stored and do not last long. Each person's appetite helps him or her choose the quality of food to eat. If a person is healthy, he or she will choose the food necessary to bring nutrient stores back to normal.

However, often, in a case of obesity, stress, and persistent low blood sugar, the normal feeding regulatory mechanism is out of order. In this case, what the appetite desires or craves is not what the system needs. While the hunger and satiety centers will not allow a person to forget about food until the nutrient stores are filled, a person craving and eating the wrong food, such as processed sugar, alcohol, white flour, enriched flour, corn syrup, sucrose, or fructose, will deplete additional nutrients during its processing. This person will probably continue to be hungry and never experience a feeling of satiety until all the many nutrient stores are filled. Even though water-soluble vitamins are not stored in the body, a certain amount is still necessary for the cells to reach a level of saturation with these vitamins before a person can feel satisfied. An example is the relationship of B vitamin deficiency with a craving for sweets.

A healthy person does not crave certain types of food but instead chooses foods that maintain nutrient stores. Because blood sugar is well regulated and maintained at a normal level like a time-release vitamin, we will not continue to think about food when short-term regulatory processes have ceased; we will not usually overeat, because it will cause discomfort.

You may say, "Yes, but I have a slow metabolism." This condition is possible and is probably caused by low blood levels of the hormone thyroxine, which is secreted by the thyroid gland. Decreased blood levels of thyroxine may be caused by a thyroid gland fatigued from processing too much refined sugar. The thyroid gland may also be fatigued from work overload when it fills in for an exhausted adrenal gland due to someone's never-ending stress.

Body Shape & Endocrine System Connection

The whole endocrine system, which consists of ductless glands that secrete hormones into the bloodstream, is important in the promotion and distribution of muscle and adipose tissue in the body. Testosterone, the male hormone, promotes the growth of muscle. Estrogen, the female hormone, promotes the development of fat. If the endocrine, or hormonal, system is in balance, the glands will secrete appropriate amounts of hormones to produce a well-balanced and proportioned body shape.

"At its best," my teacher, Master Pilates teacher Ron Fletcher, said, "each and every body is beautiful." However, if the hormonal system is out of balance, a disproportioned shape will result. If the thyroid gland is overstimulated, a person will balloon around the middle and remain slim in their arms and legs. An overactive adrenal gland will cause a person to thicken all over with excess weight to the front in a potbelly, a flat rear, and less weight gain in the legs. Fatigued ovary glands cause the body's excess fat to accumulate on the thighs and buttocks in a pear-shaped appearance. Extra pounds in the typical "baby fat," all-over distribution of fat on hands, arms, back, chest, stomach, hips, thighs, and rear are caused by an overworked pituitary gland.

Certain foods stimulate these glands, such as sugar and starch for the thyroid, meat and salt for the adrenals, spices and fats for the sex glands, and dairy foods for the pituitary. Only a balanced diet minimizing the stimulating foods will allow the overactive glands to rest and recover while the other glands take over more of the load of directing chemical reactions in the body. In this way, the endocrine system will have healthy glands functioning in a balanced system, producing a well-proportioned body.

What can cause the hormonal system to get out of balance? Continued chronic stress. Stress is caused by life's events. The body needs a certain amount of stress to stay healthy, but an overload of stress causes many physiological problems, including weight gain.

Excess weight in the form of fluid retention and fat serves as protection from emotions that are difficult to acknowledge. This is partly due to the hormone cortisol. Cortisol (as well as corticosteroids and prednisone) is secreted in excess when we are under chronic stress, resulting in fluid retention and weight gain.

We're all aware of stress being a factor in heart disease or stomach ulcers. Stress has many forms, good and bad — work overload, not enough rest, new job, new home, marriage, pregnancy and childbirth, death of a loved one, divorce, illness, or any other emotional crisis. No matter what the cause, the body reacts to stress in the same primitive "fight-or-flight" response that was meant to be a temporary action for survival. If a person did not win the fight or flee from danger, his or her life was ended.

While a little stress is necessary for life, too much stress is destructive. Stress increases the body's functions, such as heart rate and blood pressure. This causes a much greater demand for the body's nutrients, causing a decrease in energy stores, which in extreme cases become completely depleted. During stressful situations, extra care should be taken to ensure that adequate nutrients are made available to replenish the nutrient storage depots.

Another Perspective on Body Types & Weight Gain

From the many students I have seen in my classes, I believe there is a connection between body shapes, hormone levels, and the foods we eat.

A pattern in patients' hormone levels is explained in the book *The Body Shaping Diet* by Sandra Cabot (Castrone). Four body type categories are described: Thyroid, Android,

Gynaeoid, and Lymphatic. Thyroid patients were small in size with low hormone levels, low blood sugar levels, and a tendency toward nervous disorders. Android patients were apple-shaped and produced lots of male androgens. Gynae-oid patients were pear-shaped and produced a high quantity of female estrogen. Lymphatic patients were straight-up-and-down-shaped with a sluggish lymph system.

The book suggests weight gain happens for four reasons: our metabolism slows down as we age; we eat to satisfy emotional hunger; we are taking inappropriate hormones; or we are on the wrong diets for our individual body shapes.

In the book *Atlas of Men,* William Herbert Sheldon describes body types after three fundamental elements of embryonic development: endoderm, mesoderm, and ectoderm. Supposedly, the individual's mental characteristics are related to his or her body. The ectomorph physique is slim and has long, thin muscles and limbs, with a low ability to store fat or build muscle. Mesomorph physique has medium-size bones, a muscular torso, low fat levels, wide shoulders, and a narrow waist, with the ability to build muscle but not to store fat. Endomorph physique characteristics are increased fat storage, a wide waist, and large bone structure.

The idea that these general body types may correlate with psychological types resembles ideas found within the concept of Ayurveda.

Ayurveda, a science of self-healing, originated in India around 3000 BC. The fundamental principles of Ayurveda were discovered by ancient Rishis, "seers of truth." They were the same Rishis who developed India's original systems of yoga and meditation. Collectively, all of these systems are known as Vedic science. Ayurveda spread with Vedic and Hindu culture to many parts of the world and is thought to have influenced ancient Greek medicine.

A central principle of Ayurveda is that there are three fundamental energy-operating forces (doshas): air, fire, and water, which regulate life in all plant and animal forms. The Vata dosha is air, the Pitta is fire, and the Kapha is water. According to Ayurveda, we are each born with a unique mixture of the Vata, Pitta, and Kapha doshas, which influences our physical and mental characteristics, including body shape, body weight, and temperament.

People of Vata constitution are generally thin physically and underdeveloped, with visible veins and muscle tendons. People of medium height and moderate body weight and muscle development have Pitta constitution. They may show a medium prominence of veins and muscle tendons. People of Kapha constitution have well-developed bodies and a strong tendency to carry excess weight. Veins and tendons are not obvious due to their thick skin and good muscle development.

Your inborn constitution represents your balanced state of health. If your present ratio of doshas does not match your constitution, you are out of balance and may be experiencing some degree of poor health. Conditions that affect the balance of doshas come from food, odors, noises, climate, and emotional states.

During the 5,000 years of Ayurveda's development, all types of foods have been analyzed for their effect on the balance of our doshas. It has been found that the way a food influences our doshas is largely a matter of its taste. During the time Ayurveda was developing, there was no knowledge of vitamins, minerals, carbohydrates, proteins, or fats. Ayurveda categorizes tastes into six types: sweet, sour, salty, bitter, pungent, and astringent.

To maintain balanced doshas and health, Ayurveda recommends including at least a little of all six tastes in your daily food intake. Even if you are trying to bring one of the doshas back into balance by eating foods with tastes that balance that dosha, you should still try to include the other tastes in your daily meals.

Ayurveda grew as practitioners of the science made very meticulous observations of human beings and the natural world. Ayurveda is practiced today as a medical science in India and other parts of the Eastern world. A recent interest among Western physicians is part of a renewed inquiry into methods of preventative, holistic, and cost-effective systems of health care.

Additional information, along with a self-test that allows you to get a general idea of your individual constitution, can be found in *The Quick & Easy Ayurvedic Cookbook* by Eileen Keavy Smity. Your highest-scoring dosha is your dominant dosha. Many people have two high-scoring doshas, which means both doshas dominate. It is rare for all three doshas to have almost the same score.

According to Ayurveda, maintenance of a proper diet along with exercise is fundamental to an individual's ability to remain healthy and in shape. The diet should be chosen to suit each individual's constitution.

A similarity is found in the three different body shapes given different labels by different generations and cultures. Foods that are helpful for one person could be harmful for another. Once you evaluate which constitution your body fits, you can choose a diet to suit your needs. Even though you may have a craving for a food that is not the best for your overall health, remember "mind over matter, or matter won't mind."

A Popular Habit Ayurveda Prohibits

A popular activity today that Ayurveda does not recommend is chewing gum. All the chewing with nothing to digest aggravates agni, the digestive fire which consists of digestive acids and enzymes that break down all the foods you eat.

A state of health exists when agni is in a balanced state, Vata-Pitta-Kapha are in equilibrium, waste products (urine, feces, and sweat) are normal, the senses function normally, and the body, mind, consciousness all work together as one. If any one of these systems is disturbed, the disease process begins. Gum chewing, with its disturbance of agni, leads to digestive disorders, which are the common source of nearly all disorders, according to Ayurveda. The only healthy time to chew gum is after you have finished eating, because you already have food in your stomach to digest.

HEALTH PROBLEMS

Some health problems will not be solved by cardiovascular endurance, strength, flexibility, good body mechanics, and nutrition. The next section provides additional self-help information for you.

Liver & Gallbladder Flush

Staying healthy includes balanced body alignment along with maintaining healthy organs and glands. While reading the book *The Amazing Liver & Gallbladder Flush*, I gained important information about the liver, our largest organ. Andres Moritz, the author, described how our liver is involved in numerous essential body functions to maintain the growth and function of every cell in our body. He listed many symptoms that were probably caused by numerous gallstones in the liver and gallbladder. He also included a process on how to keep the liver healthy.

The liver produces cholesterol, hormones, bile, amino acids, and proteins; filters our blood and recycles proteins from old cells; and is linked to all parts of the body, including the nervous and endocrine systems. After bile is produced in the liver, it passes from the liver through bile ducts into the gallbladder, pancreas, and small intestine. Health problems begin to occur when a congestion of gallstones in the bile ducts suffocates healthy cells and blocks pathways of circulation, as well as the elimination of toxins and waste matter, causing a detrimental impact on the health of our whole body.

After reading the book, I decided to follow the liver-gallbladder flush process. Years before, I was advised to do a flush by Ayurvedic and homeopathic practitioners. Since I had no symptoms that I might have gallstones, it was a surprise that by the time I completed the flush, I had eliminated over two hundred and forty gallstones.

Our body processes bacteria, parasites, and wastes into a form that can be removed from our body. If bile ducts are congested with gallstones, another line of defense is mucus. Mucus secretions in the chest and nasal passages will trap toxins so that they can be removed. I had an experience that had never happened before—congestion in my chest and nasal passages for five months. My holistic wellness doctor found that bacteria and a virus were in my spleen. I believe that if I had practiced an annual liver-gallbladder flush, gallstones would not have blocked bile, which is important to the immune system, and a natural, healthy process of removing toxins from my system would have occurred.

A relative had a severe gallbladder condition. Early one morning, he experienced pain in his pelvis. Never before had he experienced such pain. He went to his doctor, and his blood test showed a very high white blood cell count, which indicated an infection. He was scheduled to have an ultrasound test the next day, but later that day, the pain had increased so severely that he went to the hospital's emergency room. His gallbladder had ruptured and had to be removed. Evidently, it can take up to eight years before noticeable gallstone symptoms occur. Perhaps an annual liver-gallbladder flush would have prevented his experience.

Hearing Loss

I have always been concerned about hearing loss. When I was an infant, my father was in an automobile accident and suffered a head injury that damaged his inner ear and hearing. He could hear, but sound coming into his hearing-damaged side was minimal. From an early age, I was able to witness the challenges of living with hearing loss.

Usually, hearing loss is caused by damage to the inner ear from aging or prolonged exposure to loud noise. The process of hearing occurs when sound waves pass through the outer ear and create sound waves at the eardrum. The eardrum and small bones of the middle ear amplify the vibrations as they travel to the inner ear. Within the inner ear, vibrations pass through fluid and thousands of tiny hair/nerve cells that translate sound vibrations into electrical signals, which are transmitted to the brain. Regular exposure to loud sounds causes damage to the hair/nerve cells. When this happens, electrical signals from the brain are not transmitted as efficiently as healthy cells and it eventually leads to permanent hearing loss.

With many people of all ages worldwide using cell phones, iPods, iPads, etc., and hands-free accessories, unless they keep their volume at a healthy level, more people will experience hearing loss from inner ear cell damage before they would experience it from the aging process *(fig. 1)*.

Other causes of hearing loss are earwax and swimmer's ear. If the head is not in a level, balanced position, earwax may build up rather than drain out. At a certain point, the earwax will block the ear canal, preventing the conduction of sound waves to the inner ear and causing hearing loss. After swimming, if a swimmer's head is not held in a level position, water may remain in the ear rather than drain out. The water breaks down the skin and provides a breeding ground for bacteria, leading to an infection of the ear canal.

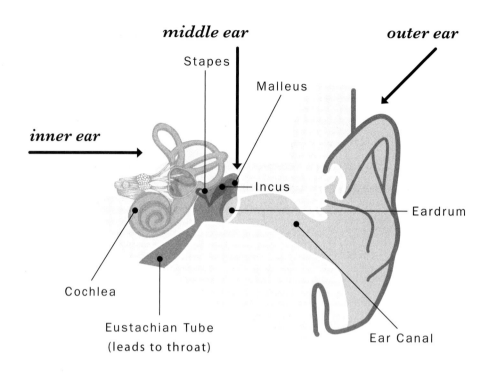

inner ear

middle ear

outer ear

Stapes

Malleus

Incus

Eardrum

Cochlea

Eustachian Tube
(leads to throat)

Ear Canal

hearing cells

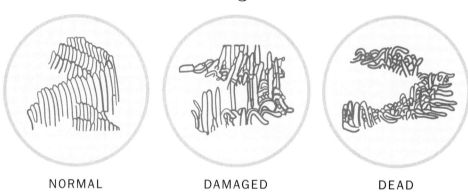

NORMAL

DAMAGED

DEAD

FIGURE 1

damaged & dead hearing cells

*Hearing hair cells in your inner ear are responsible for
sending sound impulses to the brain.*

Carpal Tunnel Syndrome & Vitamin B6

In the 1980s, I was not aware of carpal tunnel syndrome until two of my Dailey Inner Core Workout students told me they had carpal tunnel syndrome. One student was pregnant, and the other had arthritis.

I researched and found an article at UT Southwestern Medical Center Library about a research study on the connection between vitamin B deficiency and carpal tunnel syndrome. The research scientists were from Texas, so I was able to contact one of the scientists, Dr. John M. Ellis, by phone. We discussed my students' situation, and he sent me a copy of the research study.

Unlike oil-soluble vitamins that are stored in body cells, vitamin B is water soluble and cannot be stored. It must be replenished regularly through foods and supplements, if necessary. Conditions such as pregnancy, arthritis, diabetes, and others increase the need for pyridoxine, vitamin B6. When there is a vitamin B6 deficiency, cushion cells that protect the median nerve in the carpal tunnel of the hand begin to melt away and pain begins to be felt. Cell protection for the nerves is similar to rubber protection for electrical wires. With vitamin B6 supplements, correction of the deficiency in the number of cellular molecules of cushion protection for the nerves takes up to three months. Also, it is always good to include a complete B complex in addition to the extra B6 for therapeutic results.

The study also noted that there was a connection between vitamin B6 deficiency and the use of birth control pills. Since I had been taking the pills at that time, I changed my diet to natural, whole-grain foods and added B vitamins to my regimen.

I learned of another effect of vitamin B deficiency for myself. I have always had a "sweet tooth" but was satisfied with one serving of dessert. In the 1980s, I became addicted to sweets. When I read this study and began to take B vitamins, the cravings began to decrease. After three months, my sweet tooth was back to normal, and my vitamin B levels were satisfied.

Macular Degeneration & Nutrition

Dr. Conrad Speece, my osteopathic doctor, told me about the healing experience of one of his patients. She was diagnosed with macular degeneration by her full-time ophthalmologist, who was teaching at the University of Texas Southwestern Medical Center. He then sent her to a retina specialist, who confirmed the diagnosis. She did not know what having macular degeneration meant, so she called back her ophthalmologist, who was also a personal friend. She told him that the retina specialist confirmed the diagnosis. Her ophthalmologist friend told her that she would eventually go blind. She had her husband take her to Light House for the Blind, an association that provides services to help blind and visually impaired individuals. She wanted to sign up to be a volunteer and learn to read Braille.

Then a friend referred her to Dr. Ron Overberg, a licensed dietitian and clinical nutritionist with a PhD in biology. From her blood test information and symptoms of macular degeneration, Dr. Overberg prescribed a supplement program including vitamin A and carotenoid complex.

She was on the program for several weeks and continued the program when she and her husband went to visit their daughter in New England. Her granddaughter asked her to read to her one night and kept insisting. She finally picked up the book and realized that she could read to her granddaughter without her glasses.

After six weeks, when she came back home, she went to UT Southwestern for a checkup. The retina specialist tested her then called another doctor in to run the test because he thought he had made a mistake. They both concluded that her macular degeneration was gone and her eyes were better than those of most people her age. She continued on the supplement program to prevent the condition from returning.

Low Salt Intake & Health

One of the current recommendations to improve your health is to reduce your salt intake. How can this be when salt is an essential nutrient for a healthy body? Our cells live in salt water. And remember, the self-healing science of Ayurveda found that salt is one of six tastes necessary to maintain health.

When the blood level of salt (sodium) in the body becomes abnormally low, it causes a condition known as hyponaturemia. The condition may cause a person to suddenly become light-headed with a racing heart and pounding chest. Low-salt diets may increase insulin resistance. If tests show that the blood level of salt is abnormally low, a saline solution drip with sodium is prescribed. A patient feels normal when the sodium level is raised to the correct level.

According to Dr. Dong-Rae Park, OMD, an oriental medicine doctor, certain sodium levels in the blood may aggravate problems in weakened systems of the body. Since salt is an essential nutrient to the body, its reduction should be temporary while the unbalanced systems are being brought back to normal.

Certain types of salt may be medicinal. My Ayurveda doctor recommended an after-dinner drink, Digestive Lassi, to stimulate and increase digestive fire to help my digestive system. One of the ingredients was black salt powder, which is a special type of mineral salt from India. Rather than black, its color is a light, pinkish-gray color, and it has a sulfur-mineral taste similar to hard-boiled eggs. Evidence that Lassi improved my digestion appeared as a decrease in the impressions of my teeth on the edges of my tongue. These impressions are an indication of unabsorbed nutrients.

Salt is used worldwide to enhance flavors in many varieties of food. There is a difference between sea salt and regular table salt. Common table salt may be stripped of all trace minerals and may contain chemical bleaching agents. Sea salt has a natural balance of trace minerals and elements from the creation in sea water of salt crystals by the sun and wind.

Iodine is an important, nutritional essential element found in sea salt. I learned about the importance of iodine from a student. She had goiter, a thyroid condition that caused her thyroid gland to swell and become abnormally large due to iodine deficiency. She was raised in Ohio, which is within the Goiter Belt. It is an area in the Unites States where iodine levels are lower in locally grown foods due to low levels of iodine in the soil. It is also a far distance from the sea, and seafood that provides a very high intake of iodine is not plentiful. The primary function of the thyroid gland is to concentrate iodine and manganese from the blood to make the thyroid hormone, which furnishes energy to every cell in the body.

Japanese women have a very high intake of iodine due to the large amount of seaweed, also a source of iodine, in their diet. They also have very low levels of breast cancer, goiter, and hypothyroidism.

I learned about an efficient and economical method to determine the body's metabolic deficiency of iodine from Dr. Overberg. If an application of tincture of iodine to your skin fades within twenty-four hours, it indicates that your body's iodine level is not sufficient to normalize thyroid secretion to the cells.

Dr. Overberg's instructions were based on the method of application from Jean Surbeck, MD. Apply brown-colored 2 percent tincture of iodine to the upper thigh or lower abdomen in a three-inch square patch. Apply as often as you notice the iodine is absorbed and the skin is clear. When you apply one application and the stain is visible for twenty-four hours, discontinue application, as it is an indication that your iodine levels are normal.

I tested the procedure on myself. After the first application, in less than two hours, the brown stain had faded. I had no idea my iodine levels were low. It took a while, but with repeated applications, iodine was absorbed into my internal system, and the brown stain was visible after twenty-four hours. I continue to check my iodine absorption annually.

Cortisone

Cortisone inhibits the activity of fibroblasts, the sources of connective tissue. This effect of cortisone has been used pharmaceutically in the treatment of fibrosis—dense connective tissue deposits created by repeated strain in the muscle belly, the thickest part of the muscle, which is usually between the insertion and origin. This hormone also acts as an anti-inflammatory substance, and as such has been applied to inflammations of all kinds to reduce the swelling and discomforts they create. However, the negative effects of continued exposure to cortisone have revealed themselves to be substantially greater than the positive effects in the long run.

Anything that depresses fibroblast activity obviously interferes with the normal healing of wounds, bruises, fractures, and the like, no matter how effectively it reduces the swelling associated with these injuries. Neither has cortisone proved to be as useful in the treatment of infections and inflammatory allergic reactions as was once hoped; it simply removes discomforting symptoms without affecting either the basic mechanism or the cause of the infection. In fact, since it weakens the connective tissue, it has been shown to actually facilitate the spread of infection from previously localized areas. Animals that have been given large amounts of cortisone develop spontaneous and rapidly fatal infections.

I learned about the negative effects of continued exposure of cortisone when my cat had a urinary tract infection. The veterinarian gave her a cortisone shot. It helped for a while, but the infection returned and the vet gave her another dose. The third time the infection returned, the vet said that due to liver damage caused from cortisone, it would be her last dose of cortisone. He would not ever give her another dose.

Health Benefits from Nutritional Supplements

Dr. Overberg told me about a seventy-year-old registered engineer who was taking medications for a variety of health issues: Cardizem for high blood pressure, Hytrin for shrinking and hardening bladder, Pamelor for ulnar nerve pain, and Zantac and Reglan for hiatal hernia. He was on an air pressure machine for sleep apnea every night, had manipulations from an osteopathic doctor for lumbar back pain and regular coal tar treatments for psoriasis, followed a low-fat diet for years but was still seventy-five to eighty-five pounds overweight, and suffered from low energy (going to bed early at night and sleeping late in the morning), but he had no procedure to heal his glaucoma and cataracts. He felt he was at his lowest level of physical health.

Then he met Dr. Overberg. After information from his blood test and a description of his symptoms, Dr. Overberg suggested nutritional supplements: Formula 4 multivitamin, premium protein, carotenoids and vitamin A for the eyes, salmon oil and lecithin for vascular problems, B complex for nerve and back problems, Betagest for reflux, Resp 11 for allergies, Doctor's Diet for weight reduction, vitamins C and E, and Men's Formula.

Two years later, he was at a point where he was no longer on pharmaceutical medications, his glaucoma was gone, his cataracts were shrinking, his blood pressure was down to 135/68 or lower, psoriasis had almost disappeared, he didn't have to sleep with a mask on his face, and he experienced no more reflux. He could feel the benefits of the supplements Dr. Overberg had prescribed, and they made a tremendous change in his life. He was ready to celebrate his seventy-second birthday.

More information on the nutritional supplements can be found at www.gnld.com.

Side Effects of Medicines

A woman who had sudden and severe tightness in the chest, dizziness, and nausea thought she was having a heart attack. After going to the emergency room, having tests for two days at the hospital, and receiving no answers, she later discovered the cause—unexpected side effects from a prescription drug she had started taking three weeks earlier to manage a mild thyroid condition.

This is just an example of how medications can cause other conditions unrelated to the health problems they are prescribed to treat. Unaware that almost all medications have side effects, patients will consult their doctors about the new condition, only to be prescribed another drug that could produce still more side effects.

Adverse drug effects send about 4.5 million Americans to the doctor's office or the emergency room each year—more than for common conditions like strep throat or pneumonia —according to a study by the federal Agency for Healthcare Research and Quality. The National Academy of Sciences's Institute of Medicine estimates that serious drug reactions occur more than two million times each year among patients in hospitals and are the fourth leading cause of hospital deaths, topped only by heart disease, cancer, and stroke (Barry).

Milder symptoms such as drowsiness, sleeplessness, muscle aches, dizziness, nausea, and bouts of depression may be more troubling than they are dangerous. Yet, studies show that drugs that affect people's sense of balance or slow their reactions are a major cause of falls and road accidents.

Drugs that are prescribed for a specific health problem and trigger other health problems are sometimes errors made by doctors, pharmacists, and hospitals. Even if all errors are avoided, issues remain, including bad interactions among different drugs prescribed for the same patient by different doctors, drugs prescribed for uses that the Food and Drug Administration has not approved, and an imperfect testing system for new drugs, which permits the marketing of medications that later prove to have harmful side effects.

More than 75 percent of Americans age sixty and over take two or more prescription drugs, and 37 percent use at least five, according to the federal Centers for Disease Control and Prevention. However, older people are rarely included in clinical trials, which test a drug's safety and effectiveness.

Drug manufacturers recommend that doctors prescribe and that patients buy the newest, most expensive medications. But studies show that six out of seven "new" drugs are no more effective than "old" ones, and they are riskier because they haven't been around long enough to have an extensive safety record. Many doctors are becoming more conservative, prescribing fewer prescription drugs and lower dosages.

From a patient's perspective, it's easier to take a pill a day rather than to diet or exercise. It is also easier for physicians to prescribe pills, especially when people tend to want their money's worth when making an office visit.

It is not always easy to tell whether a symptom is related to a drug, a drug interaction, the underlying medical condition, or a different health problem entirely. If a drug is suspected, the only way a doctor can be certain it's the cause is to stop prescribing the drug and see if the symptom vanishes. This might be medically feasible for some conditions but not others.

CANCER & OXYGEN

I gained an insight about cancer at a reunion from a college roommate who had majored in biology. After graduation, she worked for an MD/oncologist in his research lab. He told her that we all have at least 140 cancer cells in our body. This is common knowledge to scientists, but not to the majority of the population, including myself. When I mentioned the cancer cell information to my teacher, she showed me a book she had been reading, *Cancer Is Not a Disease—It's a Survival Mechanism*, by Andreas Moritz. I was so curious that I immediately read the book.

Moritz, a practitioner of Ayurveda, states in his book that cancer cells are anaerobic, meaning they cannot survive in oxygen. Cancer cells live in an anaerobic environment, breaking down waste materials, toxic deposits, and dead, worn-out cells. When there is a continued drastic deprivation of vital nutrients, including oxygen, to healthy cells, some of the cells will die, but others mutate into cancer cells. Thus the cells converted to cancer are able to live without oxygen and will get their energy from metabolic waste.

Moritz interviewed many cancer patients and found that almost all cancer survivors shared one experience: The disease caused the most important and positive changes in their lives. He also found that during their battle with cancer, almost all patients felt burdened by some sort of stress: constant conflicts, resentment, guilt, shame, poor self-image, unresolved conflict, worries, or past emotional uneasiness.

The fight-or-flight response that occurs when one is under stress or feels threatened prevents the body from being able to utilize its maximum healing capacity. Our amounts and duration of stress have greatly increased since ancient times, when a fight or flight would continue only until there was a win, escape, or the end.

Cancer seems to be turning into an epidemic. I asked my DO what he thought about the relationship of stress and cancer. He estimated that three years after the 2008 economic downturn, there would be a major increase in cancer patients due to stress.

I have noticed that some of my students carry tension in muscles of their shoulders, neck, feet, jaws, wrists, and more. Tight muscles decrease blood circulation to the area of muscle tension. From one person, I learned that his posture may have contributed to the kidney cancer spreading to his spine. The doctor said his kidneys were compressing against his spine, blocking blood circulation, nutrients, oxygen, and life force. His standing posture was with his pelvis tilted backward, tailbone tucked under (sad-dog tail). This also made me wonder how posture might affect reproductive organ problems: sad-dog tail for men and rooster tail for women. It is essential to maintain balanced body alignment for good health, our most valuable asset.

The Power of Posture

When you walk into a room and look around, for better or worse, before you even open your mouth, you have made an impression, and posture is one of the first traits people notice. Fifty percent of the impression we make is based on our body language. Research has shown that people are influenced more by body language than by verbal language. We, as do other mammals, communicate our feelings through our posture. For example, it is easy to see that a dog feels sad when its head and tail are tucked under.

The origins of poor posture are often deeply rooted. Our attitudes and emotions are reflected in our body language. An emotional trauma causing anger or fear may lead to protective, tense, muscular body armor. It may be linked to adolescence, when girls self-consciously stoop to hide developing bodies. If poor posture becomes habitual, our joints will become stiff and our muscles will lose some of their flexibility and strength. Slumped posture may also invite threatening approaches from others. In the wild, predators attack the weakest animals or plants.

However, every group of animals has an alpha leader whose posture is strong, upright, and assertive. Alpha posture is helpful to us in communicating to our children, employees, and associates. With an awareness of our posture, the components of balanced alignment and alpha posture, we can create more positive social encounters *(figs. 2–6)*.

Good upright posture can promote an aura of confidence. Posture also affects your positive mental attitude (PMA). A person with alpha posture tends to have a balanced emotional state and a positive attitude. Without tension in the muscles of the neck and shoulders, oxygenation to the brain increases. When the muscles of your neck are balanced and your "head is on straight," your mind can think more clearly.

Body chemistry is also affected by balanced postural alignment, which provides a healthy flow of blood to organs and glands. Hormones of the endocrine system, including those that regulate fat metabolism, reproduction, and sexual health, are balanced. Alpha posture also has beneficial effects on other body systems, which include respiratory, musculoskeletal, digestive, elimination, and immune systems.

On the other hand, unbalanced posture could possibly contribute to a common respiratory system problem, asthma. A neighbor whose son had asthma was told by his doctor that the usual posture for patients with asthma was a posterior

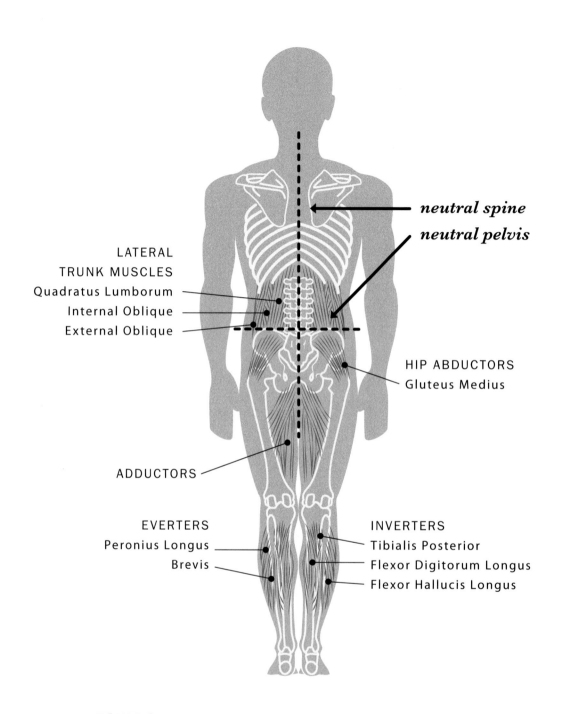

LATERAL
TRUNK MUSCLES
Quadratus Lumborum
Internal Oblique
External Oblique

neutral spine
neutral pelvis

HIP ABDUCTORS
Gluteus Medius

ADDUCTORS

EVERTERS
Peronius Longus
Brevis

INVERTERS
Tibialis Posterior
Flexor Digitorum Longus
Flexor Hallucis Longus

FIGURE 2

ideal alignment: posterior view

All muscles are balanced.

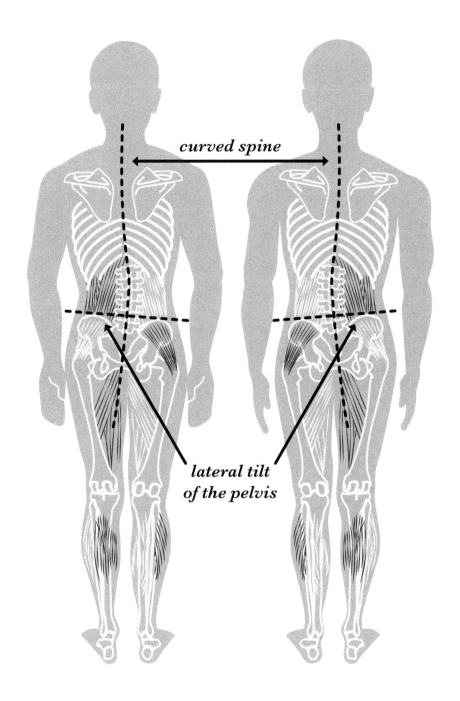

FIGURE 3

faulty alignment: lateral tilt

Lighter lines represent elongated and weak muscles.

Darker lines represent short and strong muscles.

tilted pelvis (sad-dog tail) *(fig. 5)* with slumped chest, round-ed shoulders, and forward head position. The respiratory ca-pacity of this type of body alignment is greatly reduced.

Studies have shown that when you are in a bad mood, if you stand up straight, open your eyes widely, and put a smile on your face, your PMA will improve. It will also im-prove other people's perception of you—giving you an im-pression of approachability and confidence. Sometimes you have to "fake it 'til you make it," just as when a theater per-former is on stage and must portray a specific emotion.

Alpha shoulder posture *(figs. 2 and 4)* balances muscles on the front (anterior) side of the shoulder girdle with those on the back (posterior) side. The breastbone lifts and the ribs open outward, providing more space for the lungs. This im-proves respiration, induces relaxation, and strengthens the immune system. It lowers heart rate and blood pressure, as shown by research studies on yoga and heart disease by Dr. Dean Ornish. Strengthened back muscles also help to pre-vent kyphosis, the hump between shoulder blades, and for-ward head position, decreasing the possibility of having ten-sion headaches.

An alpha posture levels and balances your pelvic girdle, thus giving all the visceral organs the space to function effi-ciently. Digestion and elimination are improved. With bal-anced pelvic girdle muscles, the hips are narrowed, stomach is flattened, thighs are toned, and lower back is lengthened and strengthened, decreasing your risk of injury and back pain.

The musculoskeletal system benefits greatly from alpha shoulder and pelvic girdle posture. It decreases muscle and joint strain and loss of height, promotes efficient movement, and provides an aesthetic physical appearance. After adopt-ing this new posture, one student told me, "I have greatly improved my posture and lost a size in clothing . . . not to mention generally feeling energized and better overall."

FIGURE 4

ideal alignment: side view

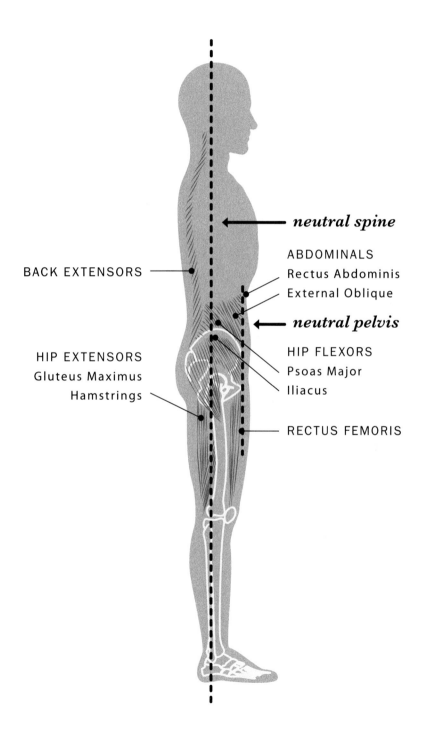

neutral spine

ABDOMINALS
Rectus Abdominis
External Oblique

neutral pelvis

BACK EXTENSORS

HIP FLEXORS
Psoas Major
Iliacus

HIP EXTENSORS
Gluteus Maximus
Hamstrings

RECTUS FEMORIS

FIGURE 5

faulty alignment: posterior tilt

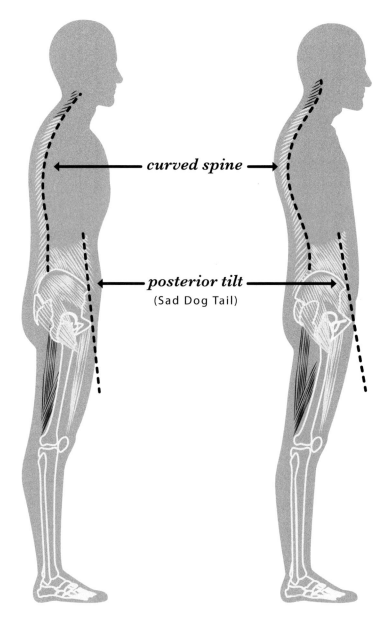

curved spine

posterior tilt
(Sad Dog Tail)

FLAT-BACK POSTURE   SWAY-BACK POSTURE

FIGURE 6
faulty alignment: anterior tilt

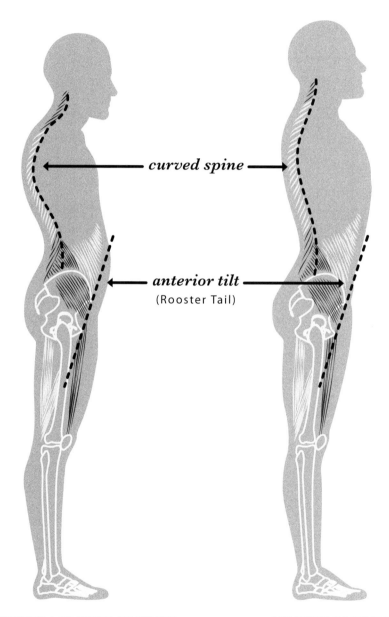

KYPHOTIC LORDOTIC POSTURE   MILITARY POSTURE

The mind and emotions have an important influence on the development, shape, and health of the body. Conversely, the body has an equally important influence on the health and development of the mind and emotions. The body stores tension from its experiences. If you have experienced much trauma or abuse, chronic tension will be locked in as body armor. The tension will create an imbalance in muscle pairs that will eventually result in discomfort and pain. Through corrective exercises, tension will slowly dissolve. When tension release occurs, emotions that caused the tension may also be released—as though the body is the key to the subconscious mind. One of my students would schedule counseling appointments after Dailey Inner Core Workout classes in order to process emotions released following the movements.

Toxins stored in tense muscles will also be released. The sudden release of toxins into the circulatory system may cause nausea. In extreme cases, it may cause regurgitation and diarrhea.

The first step to developing better posture and an intelligent body is to create an awareness of your body alignment and participate in Dailey Inner Core Workout. The Workout will provide movements that reprogram unbalanced muscles. Regular participation in these movements will equalize strength with flexibility between your muscle pairs, which will give you broad shoulders and lower back ribs, narrow hips, and a lengthened spine. Your shoulders, hips, and spine must work together: your neck vertebrae will not lengthen and center your head unless your shoulders are open and broad; your lumbar spine (back of the waist) will not lengthen unless your hips are narrowed; your hips will not narrow unless your feet are in parallel position with your toes together and heels apart. With unified action in all areas of your body, you will reap the benefits of alpha posture.

Respiration

At birth, newborns must quickly make physiological adjust-
ments so that they can do for themselves those things that
their mothers' bodies had been doing for them in the womb.
When the fetus is forced through the birth canal and cervix
to leave the mother's body (removing fluid as it goes and
leaving a vacuum in its lungs), the most immediate need is to
receive oxygen. The first breath must be particularly forceful
because the newborn's lungs are collapsed and the airways
are small and offer considerable resistance to air movement.

Fortunately, the lungs of a full-term fetus secrete surfac-
tant, which reduces surface tension within the alveoli (air
sacs of the lungs). After the newborn takes its first powerful
breath, the lungs begin to expand and breathing becomes
easier.

If the newborn had the umbilical cord wrapped around
its neck or was born during a caesarean procedure, it had a
totally different birth experience and as an adult will usually
have less respiratory capacity than an adult of vaginal birth.
Also, the nares (nostril openings) of people born by caesarean section are smaller than those of natural birth, and they
are not able to intake as much breath.

The two nostrils of the nose provide openings through
which air can enter and exit the nasal cavity. The nasal cavity, a hollow space behind the nose, is divided in the middle
into right and left portions. On each side, the cavity is divided into three nasal passageways: superior meatus, middle
meatus, and inferior meatus. They conduct the air from the
nasal cavity through the larynx and trachea into the lungs
(*fig. 7*).

The superior meatus passage directs breath to the lowest
part of the lungs. The inferior surfaces of the lungs are attached to the superior surface of the diaphragm. By contract-
ing the diaphragm muscle along with relaxed low abdominal

muscles, volume of the lungs increases and causes air to enter the lungs for inspiration, similar to blowing up a balloon. This is a deep-cleansing type of breathing used in the practice of yoga. To help direct your breath to the lower lungs during inspiration, imagine breathing behind your eyes to your low lungs, and feel your low abdominals relax. This increases the volume of your lungs as they move toward your pelvis and swell your lower abdomen.

The middle meatus passage is located inside the middle of your nose (where athletes place nasal strips on the nose surface to help improve nasal breathing by reducing nasal airflow resistance). Inhalation through the middle meatus directs the breath to the mid-area of your lungs. The low ribs expand equally all around, like a bellows, allowing the abdominal muscles to support your lower back while you are active. When people aren't aware of how they are breathing, they often expand the anterior ribs, increasing the lumbar arch, tightening lower back muscles and weakening their core abdominal muscles.

The inferior meatus directs breath to your upper lung at the clavicles, or collarbones. Imagine smelling a rose. If your head is level, you will feel the breath directed behind your clavicles, relaxing and lengthening muscles of your neck and head.

Respiration is such a strong instinct that we often are not aware of how the process works (*figs. 7–8*). The number of muscles involved in regular versus forced inspiration and expiration will amaze you. There is only one muscle in your body with the sole purpose of helping you breathe, and that is the diaphragm. I gained this information about the muscles we use to breathe during my studies for an MS in exercise physiology. Take a look:

> *Inspiration:* diaphragm, intercostals, levatores costarum (three muscles used)

FIGURE 7

respiratory system

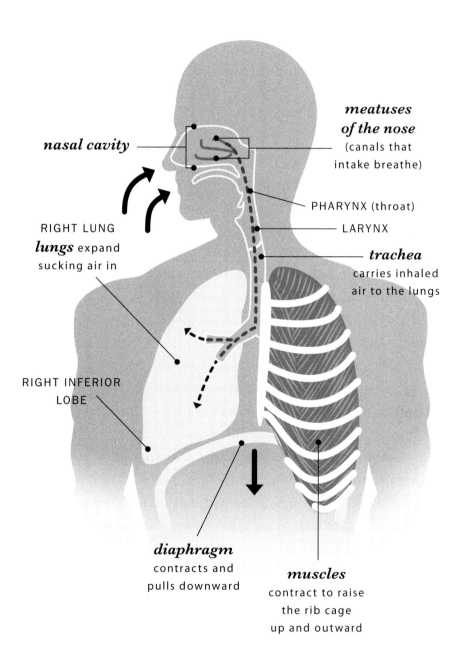

*meatuses
of the nose*
(canals that
intake breathe)

nasal cavity

PHARYNX (throat)

LARYNX

trachea
carries inhaled
air to the lungs

RIGHT LUNG
lungs expand
sucking air in

RIGHT INFERIOR
LOBE

diaphragm
contracts and
pulls downward

muscles
contract to raise
the rib cage
up and outward

FIGURE 8

respiration

inhalation   *exhalation*

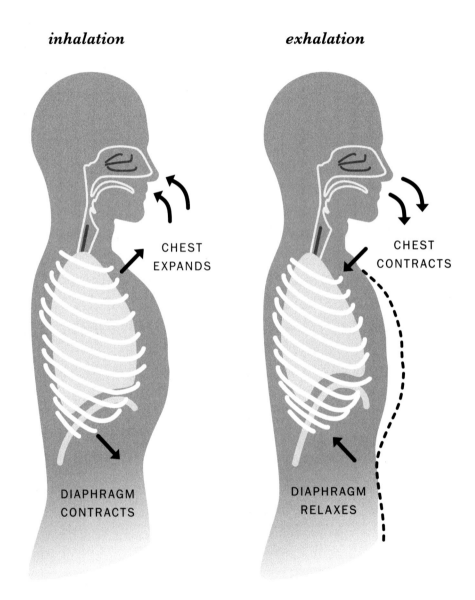

CHEST
EXPANDS

DIAPHRAGM
CONTRACTS

CHEST
CONTRACTS

DIAPHRAGM
RELAXES

> *Expiration:* transversus thoracis, rectus abdominis, transversus abdominis, obliquus externus, obliquus internus, pyramidalis (six muscles used)

> *Forced Inspiration:* diaphragm, intercostales, levatores costarum, subcostales, sternocleidomastoideus, semispinalis, spinalis, multifidus, rotatores, interspinales, scalenus anterior, scalenus medius, scalenus posterior, subclavius, serratus anterior, pectoralis major, pectoralis minor, serratus posterior superior (eighteen muscles used)

> *Forced Expiration:* transversus thoracis, rectus abdominis, transversus abdominis, obliquus externus, obliquus internus, pyramidalis, longissimus dorsus, iliocostalis, latissimus dorasi, serratus posterior inferior, quadratus lumborum, coccygeus, levator ani, transversus perinei superficialis, transversus perinei profundus (fifteen muscles used)

There's a good reason why so many muscles work together to help you breathe: a strong respiratory capacity is essential to your good health, and cardiovascular activities are necessary to maintain respiratory capacity. Interestingly enough, two professions are credited with enjoying the longest lifespans—orchestra conductors and horse jockeys. Some people have speculated that the health secret of conductors Leopold Stokowski (ninety-five), Pablo Casals (ninety-six) and Nadia Boulanger (ninety) is classical music. If that were true, those who just listen would enjoy the same benefits, which isn't the case. Physicist/nutritionist/kinesiologist, Steven Rachlitz, PhD, believes that their remarkable longevity comes from a lifetime of superior cardiovascular health due to the vigorous upper body movements that define a conductor's work.

When conducting an orchestra, a conductor's arms are always in motion, most often at shoulder level or above.

These movements expand muscles of the lungs and chest. Similarly, a horse jockey rides leaning forward, holding the reins above his shoulders. This causes the muscles of the lungs and the chest to expand. Their entire body experiences more efficient oxygenation and circulation. This supports the pumping action of the heart and helps send the flow of blood, oxygen, and nutrients directly to muscles and internal organs. Having a passion for their profession and enjoying their work/play time is another health benefit for conductors and jockeys.

Contrast the activities related to these two professions to the way most of us spend our days—elbows below shoulder level, hunched over at our desks, in front of computers, or on the phone. Add the hours we spend in cars or trains, watching TV, or curled up in a chair reading. Our chests are contracted, and our breathing is shallow, inhibiting the oxygenation and circulation of our blood.

Our respiratory system also plays a very important part in the elimination of metabolic waste. Respiration removes 70 percent of the body's metabolic waste. Perspiration removes 19 percent, urination removes 8 percent, and defecation removes 3 percent. The body's respiratory capacity reaches its peak in our mid-twenties. If we do not continue to be physically active, the loss of respiratory functions could be 9 percent to 25 percent every ten years. With heart disease one of the top causes of death in people over age fifty-five, you must counter the effects of immobility on your lungs, heart, and upper body to avoid SDS (sedentary death syndrome).

Taking deep breaths and singing make you feel good. Of course, to sing properly, you must breathe deeply and stand with your posture balanced, a recipe to make you feel good naturally. Unfortunately, people sometimes choose unhealthier ways to feel good, such as smoking, alcohol, drugs, etc., but these provide only temporary feelings of satisfaction.

The pursuit of that high feeling leads from one addiction to another, yet people don't realize that the problem they really need to address is spiritual (in the spirit, inspiration). Learning to breathe deeply could allow their bodies to relax, release all stress, and give them the natural high feeling for which they are striving.

It never occurred to me that someone would smoke a cigarette to be able to breathe deeper. A young man of nineteen worked for me part-time as a temporary employee. After working several months, he took a break and went outside to smoke a cigarette. When I asked him what made him want to start smoking, he told me a friend said it helped him breathe deeper. Many people at his NA (Narcotics Anonymous) meetings were smokers, so he tried it. After investigating further, I learned that my employee was a twin, born by cesarean section two months premature, and he had been in the hospital and on a respirator for two months.

Others have said they smoked to help themselves breathe deeper. I have noticed many students begin to yawn when they focus on opening their collarbones and bringing their shoulders into balanced alignment. I witnessed an extreme example of another student who smoked and had rounded shoulder and forward-head posture. During her first lesson, when she was lying on her back in supine position on the exercise mat with her shoulders open, neck long with the back of her head on the mat, her chest opened immensely, providing more space within her lungs for inspiration. To fill the vacuum, she yawned at least forty times! Perhaps if those who attend addiction meetings practiced movements with a focus on balanced body alignment and breathing, along with the "higher power," their addiction problems would be solved.

The Influence of Mind over Matter

All of us would be in better shape if we had better posture and an attitude that promoted a better posture. A lengthened spine with all body parts brought into proper alignment adds inches to your height and takes years from your body.

One cause of developing poor posture is the force of gravity that relentlessly presses down upon us. If we are not aware of the decline of our balanced alignment, the muscles required for balanced body alignment begin to atrophy and weaken from disuse. Stress from life's events may change our body language from alpha to protective, and this is where the influence of the mind over matter comes in.

In a classic book, *Body and Mature Behavior* by Moshe Feldenkraise, the author states that immature behavior and negative emotions appear to demand flexion for emotional security. You have probably seen a shy or insecure person with rounded shoulders and a ducked head. This person feels safe and protected with this stance. Changing your posture is difficult not only because you have to change your posture itself, but also the attitude that produces the posture. A person must stand up straight to feel more secure and feel secure enough to stand up straight. A change in posture must be accompanied by a change in personality or attitude.

The Beginning of the Mind-Body Connection

Prior to the twentieth century, traditional medicine purported that there was a separation of the central nervous system—the seat of thought, memory, and emotion—from the endocrine system, which secretes powerful hormones, and the immune system, which defends the body from microbial invasions.

Aristotle was among the first to suggest the connection between mood and health. "Soul and body, I suggest, react sympathetically upon each other," he once noted. Charles

Darwin also believed the connection was important. It was a major premise of his largely overlooked book *The Expression of the Emotions in Man and Animals*. Sir William Osler, a late nineteenth- / early twentieth-century physician described as the "father of modern medicine," once remarked, "The care of tuberculosis depends more on what the patient has in his head than what he has in his chest."

Aristotle, Darwin, and Osler form an impressive trio of observers who were struck by the apparent connection between mind and body, emotions and health. Yet at that time, the scientific tools available were unable to discern the links.

Two Americans stand out both as pioneer researchers in the mind-body field and as major figures in establishing its credibility. In a landmark study of women published in 1964, psychiatrist F. Solomon and colleague Rudolf Moos demonstrated a link between emotional conflict and the onset and course of rheumatoid arthritis. Despite a genetic predisposition, certain women did not develop the disease. The disease-free women were all emotionally healthy, had good marriages, and were not depressed or alienated. It appeared that emotional health protected them from rheumatoid arthritis. At that time, the study provoked great skepticism in the scientific community (Hall).

In the 1970s, research began on psychoneuroimmunology (PNI), an interaction between the body's psychological processes and the nervous and immune systems. The theory is that the mind resides in the body as well as in the brain and emotions play an important role in disease and health. With the convergence of molecular biology, immunology, and neuroscience, scientists began to span the huge gap between emotions, mental processes, and molecules. PNI research scientists including Candace Pert, Michael Ruff, and Robert Ader began researching in detail the neuropeptides (small protein-like molecules) used by neurons (basic building blocks of the nervous system) to communicate with each other and the psychosomatic network, a network in which the mind is connected to all cells of the body as well as of the brain. The happy and sad emotions in your mind are in all of your body cells and influence the body's health and disease (Hall). Their research supports the message of Louise L. Hay in her book *Heal Your Body: The Mental Causes for Physical Illness and the Metaphysical Way to Overcome Them*.

The world's centenarians are living proof that your reality affects your health. A region of Azerbaijan near the Caspian Sea and high in the Talysh Mountains is home to one of the largest concentrations of long-lived people in the world. It is estimated that there are two hundred people of one hundred or more years of age who live in the region. They have a saying: "If you don't live to be one hundred, it is your own fault." The missteps you can make, they say, include trading the bracing mountain air for the ill winds of the lowlands, not partaking of local herbs, getting too much information, and thinking bad thoughts (Menaker).

This isn't the only location where people live to a ripe old age. The World Health Organization reported in 2001 that the people of Okinawa, Japan, are the healthiest and longest living in the world. Officials say that 427 of 1.27 million inhabitants are older than one hundred. Some of their secrets to active longevity are to have fun in their lives, take vigorous walks barefoot on a sandy Okinawan beach, join friends for morning tea before working, eat with family and friends, and have a sense of humor and purpose (Doi and Zielenziger).

Aware that sick people will absorb huge amounts of health costs, Japanese doctors are also trying to teach people to maintain a good lifestyle, which includes maintaining physical activity along with social and intellectual connectedness. Some Okinawan elders don't even need to wear glasses or hearing aids (Doi and Zielenziger).

A French woman, Jeanne Calment, lived to be 122 and was an inspiration to many. She was in good health until a month before her death. She rode a bicycle until she was one hundred, treated her skin with olive oil, and ate two pounds of chocolate a week. She gave up her two cigarettes a day and her single glass of port wine before meals when she was 117, but she still nibbled on chocolate. She had a keen sense of humor and was immune to stress. She once said, "If you can't do anything about it, don't worry about it" (Whitney).

The Importance of Healthy Feet

From long ago, people have realized the role our feet play in our overall health. The book *Reflexology: Ancient Healing Art & 21st Century Science* by Ken Orr, LMT and reflexologist, tells us that many ancient cultures (Asian, Egyptian, North American Indian, and others) used some form of foot therapy to treat disease, illnesses, and imbalances. Some type of treatment process was known in China and India as early as 5000 BC, and most historians agree that acupuncture and reflexology were later developed in China.

The acupuncture health care theory is that there are patterns of vital life force energy (chi) through the body that are essential for health. Disease is believed to be caused by disruptions of energy flow. The common treatment in acupuncture is to stimulate the energy flow body by penetration of the skin with metallic needles at a body point.

Reflexology also embraces the theory of energy and nerve pathways existing throughout our bodies. Our feet and hands are maps of our bodies, with reflex points that correspond to different body areas, organs, and glands. When energy and nerve pathways become blocked, the application of pressure in areas of the feet that connect to the organs and glands in the blocked area can induce a more uninterrupted flow of chi (energy), with improved circulation, released tension, and a return to the natural function of the affected areas of the body.

It appears that acupuncture emerged as the predominant treatment, and reflexology became largely forgotten until the Dark Ages, around 400 to 500 AD. However, remote Asian cultures in Tibet, China, and India preserved the ancient traditions. Historical evidence from about 400 BC shows images of Medicine Buddha and Buddha's footprints with carved symbols on the hands and feet.

In 1017 AD, Chinese doctor Wang Wei documented the importance of the feet in treating imbalances and disease. He often noted that the feet were the most sensitive part of the body and contained great energizing areas. During the fourteenth through sixteenth centuries, some form of foot therapy was used in Central Europe. The knowledge of Chinese energy medicine and acupuncture were not recognized by the West until 1883, when Dutch doctor Ten Tyne discovered a scientific basis for reflexology.

A young woman shared with me her story of how acupuncture was a successful treatment to unblock chi in her body. She had been unable to get pregnant for several years, and she went to see a doctor who was a fertility specialist. One day, she happened to be watching an early morning television show that featured a fertility doctor who discussed acupuncture. After hearing about a woman who had experienced infertility and had success getting pregnant following acupuncture treatments, she asked her fertility specialist what he thought about the practice. He told her several of his patients had experienced success with the treatments and to give it a try. She took his advice, had acupuncture treatments, and was successful in getting pregnant. She now has two children. Several of her friends who had fertility issues also became mothers after acupuncture treatments.

Chi needs to flow through every part of the body. Therefore, your feet and toes need to be kept healthy, so they can move with strength and flexibility. This allows the body's structural foundation to be strong and stable. Your feet are also a very important source for blood circulation. With the force of gravity, the process of getting blood circulated to the feet is easy, but how is the body able to circulate blood against gravity from your feet back up to your heart? The answer is the movement of your toes! You can feel muscles of your feet, calves, thighs, and pelvis when your toes move, lifting up and down and spreading wide.

Toes act as our second heart. If we wear shoes that bind our feet and minimize toe movement, our second heart will not be able to function well. A pointed-toe shoe may be in fashion, but do you want fashion or good health?

In addition to the feet, the knees are very important in blood circulation. Wedding planners advise wedding parties to avoid locking their knees during the wedding ceremony. If their knees are locked, blood flow returning to their heart and brain will be limited, resulting in a high probability of fainting during the ceremony.

In the long term, locking knees and the force of gravity decrease blood circulation to bones of the knee joint. The lubricating (synovial) fluid in the knee joint also dries up, causing bones to rub against each other. If oxygen, nutrients, and lubricating fluid are deprived from the knee joint for a long period of time, necrosis (death of the bone) may occur, along with a probability of the need for knee surgery. Women tend to lock their knees more than men. One proposed theory is that when women lock their knees, it places them in a protective posture and they are "standing their guard."

Corrective Change Discomfort

Everyone experiences exercise and corrective change differently. As you guide your body into balanced alignment, you may experience a sudden release of tension and muscular discomfort, or you may notice some areas of your body are resisting making the changes you are asking of it. You may even experience a corrective-change discomfort crisis. I noticed that some new students experience muscle cramps when doing a movement. Since the movement is unfamiliar to their body, rarely used muscles become fatigued and cramp. Fortunately, with a few more days of practice, the muscles grow stronger and muscle fatigue and cramps disappear.

In addition to physical responses, some students experience an emotional response from the release of muscle tension during an exercise class. Some may smile, and some may cry. The release of tension can bring back memories of an event that caused their muscles to tighten for protection.

I felt my own first corrective-change discomfort when I entered my car after a chiropractic treatment and became slightly nauseous. I told the doctor about the experience at my next appointment, and he assured me that nausea was common due to the removal of toxins. When toxins stored within tense muscles are released during a treatment, they flood the circulatory system, causing nausea. He said one of his patients had to go to the restroom due to diarrhea and vomiting after every appointment.

There is a wide range of symptoms that may occur during the course of a natural healing process. An aching body, headaches, nausea, irritability, fatigue, and other flu-type symptoms often experienced during a corrective-change crisis are primarily the effects of detoxification. The human body has a great capacity to store toxins. Eventually, they must be eliminated. The corrective-change crisis takes toxic substances out of storage and into circulation. On their way to being eliminated, these poisons cause the dramatic symptoms so often experienced.

Many doctors of chiropractic, homeopathy, or naturopathy and practitioners of other forms of holistic health believe that some diseases emerge as a result of emotional upsets, traumas, and stressful situations that unbalance the systems of the body.

Known as "The Law of Cure," a disease generally occurs from the outside of the individual and progresses inward and upward. It may begin as a skin problem on the legs and slowly progress into asthma. The symptoms resolve by progressing downward and outward in the reverse order in which they came, the most recent going away first. For this reason, many people experience a reoccurrence of old ailments, some of which may not have been evident since childhood.

Healing for a Stressed Mind & Body

We live in an impatient world. Energy from negative emotions and stress needs an appropriate expression. According to the book *Body and Mature Behavior* by Moshe Feldenkraise, negative energy is best when converted into movement; otherwise, the energy is dissipated into damage at joints, muscles, and other areas of the body.

When continual stress has caused muscles and connective tissues to shorten while muscle partners have weakened, the body may come to a place where the skeletal structure is pulled out of its natural alignment into a distorted shape. We must find a way to correct a swayed back, caved shoulders, protracting forward head, humped back, bowed legs, etc. At this point, bringing the structure back into proper alignment is very difficult.

Osteopathic, reflexology, and chiropractic treatments may be helpful in the short term, but deeper and longer-lasting results can be achieved when there is a fusion of mind and body in a movement program. If muscle tension has been present for many years, myofascial bundles without lubrication will be stuck together in a frozen position, and they will be difficult to change. It is like trying to separate two pieces of plastic wrap stuck together. Having been tight so long, muscle memory is strong and will resist change. This requires retraining in how to relax and provide myofascial (muscle and fascia, a membrane covering that separates muscle fibers, bundles, and whole muscles) release. Movements must be slow, smooth, and mindfully guided so that tight muscles will not feel threatened and react in a protective mode by adding more tension into the already tight muscles *(fig. 9)*.

The Dailey Inner Core Workout provides neuromuscular reeducation along with a stronger kinesthetic awareness, an awareness of where body parts are and what they are doing. To attain this goal, you must give constant attention to your body while performing corrective movements. Only with this kind of attention will you be able to use the body to its best advantage, to be slim and strong while moving with grace and balance.

A distorted skeletal structure can result in more problems than just an unattractive figure. Correcting structural alignment allows proper communication of the nervous system to all areas of the body. An abnormal function of cells, tissues, organs, and glands may be caused by nerve irritation produced by misaligned vertebrae. Irritated nerves can cause either decreased or increased body function in whatever organs or glands those nerves supply. For instance, a sluggish liver, gall bladder, or thyroid gland indicates decreased activity. An overactive stomach or rapid heartbeat signifies increased activity. A slow metabolism and difficulty losing weight may be a byproduct of a misaligned spine.

Maintaining good health and a youthful body shape is a multifaceted process. The weakest link is where the system begins to wear and break down. Without proper nutrition

FIGURE 9

skeletal muscle: structural layers of muscle to muscle fibers

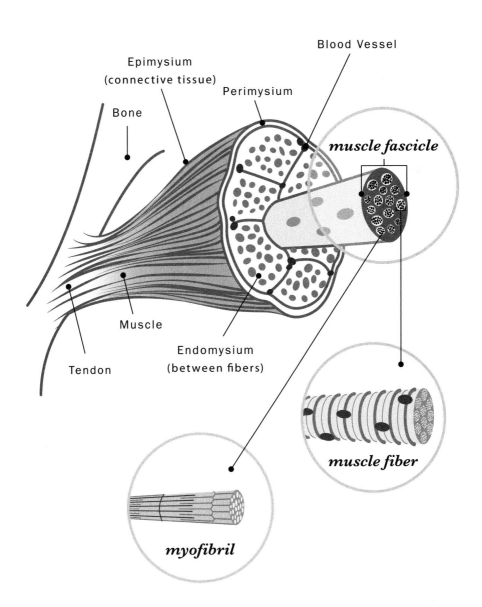

Epimysium
(connective tissue)

Perimysium

Blood Vessel

Bone

muscle fascicle

Muscle

Endomysium
(between fibers)

Tendon

muscle fiber

myofibril

and exercise of the body, mind, and spirit (the total self), the system cannot maintain itself.

We need to learn much more about the subject of health and fitness. It is arrogant to believe that we know all the answers. If we did, there would be no sickness or unfit, out-of-shape people. Our best course of action is to know ourselves and our bodies and be open to new ideas and new methods of reaching our goals.

TOO MUCH EXERCISE, TOO LITTLE EDUCATION

Are the activities of the 70s, 80s, and 90s adequate to meet the fitness needs of the Baby Boomers for the 2000s and beyond? Will these activities condition Boomers to age gracefully with few physical problems and at minimal health care expense?

The first wave of Baby Boomers reached sixty-five years of age in 2011. That year, the youngest Boomers reached middle age and were in their 40s. Those Boomers who believe in the value of exercise have participated in various aerobic activities and in strength training. Others have been involved in recreational sports, often as weekend warriors. However, unless these individuals have been taught the importance of body alignment and proper body mechanics while exercising, over time they may have developed muscular imbalances. Eventually, these imbalances will reach a level of discomfort, and, if not corrected, the next progression will lead to pain. At this point, medical advice will be required. This scenario can be prevented or corrected with education and qualified instruction in proper body alignment.

Why is body alignment so important as we age? Because it affects our most common activities: walking, standing, and sitting. It has been estimated that the average person walks the distance of two trips around the world in a lifetime. If the person's alignment is correct, each step reinforces muscular balance. Unfortunately, most people do not have correct alignment, and, in these cases, each step exacerbates muscular imbalance. Imbalances are cumulative and may not manifest themselves for years. Eventually, they may reveal themselves in various conditions, which include back, knee, and foot pain; tension headaches; shoulder tension; scoliosis; sciatica; tempo-mandibular-joint-syndrome (TMJ); and more.

Improperly performed exercise may further increase the chances of muscle imbalance. Overtraining one muscle group may pull and strain it to the point of injury. Runners frequently have such tight hip flexors that the pelvis is forced out of alignment into an exaggerated curve at the back, causing the abdominals to weaken. Without attention to abdominal strengthening combined with lower back stretching, the result will become a common complaint—back pain.

In another example, swimmers can overdevelop the pectorals in the front of the shoulder girdle, causing rounded shoulders, as well as weakness in the upper back and forward head position. In extreme cases, the anterior ribs close inward, causing a decrease in the intake of air to the lungs and swimmer's ear from the forward head position.

Another cause of muscular imbalance is due to our handedness. Out of habit, we constantly use one side of our body more than the other. We have unconscious habits like standing with more weight on one leg and always crossing the same leg over the other when sitting. Chances are we carry our shoulder bag on the same shoulder, briefcase in the same hand, and keys or wallet in the same pocket. When walking up stairs, we may lead with the same foot each time. This, taken with the possibility that there is an uneven number of stairs, may contribute to the overdevelopment of muscles on one side of the body. Even our dressing habits can cause imbalance if we continually put the same arm in our shirt sleeve or the same leg in the pant leg first, etc.

Try this simple test. Interlace your fingers. Notice which thumb in on top and which little finger is below. Now interlace your fingers with the opposite thumb on top and opposite little finger below. Does it feel awkward? Try another test. Sit tailor fashion, the way tailors used to sit on the floor and sew with their legs crossed. Reverse the position with the other leg on top. Does this position feel strange? Which hand and arm pulls the car's seat belt? We are not aware of most of our habits. All of these habits promote an imbalance of strength and flexibility of muscle pairs.

When proper stretching is not performed regularly, we create muscle imbalances. Watch infants and animals. They always stretch before moving from a resting position. They instinctively know that stretching prepares their body for movement.

If you are educated about incorrect alignment, you can make corrections from the inner core muscles and outward, saving yourself from discomfort and pain. Many physical problems that the elderly experience could be prevented or minimized by education and proper training. This would also help decrease health care costs. For example, physical therapists have found that people who have the muscle-balancing ability to squat on the floor while their feet remain flat do not have osteoarthritic knees. Their spine has maintained its embryonic curve, with balanced muscles around the knees, hips, and ankles. This means there are whole nations and millions of people who do not require knee and lower back surgery, not to mention the misery brought on by this condition. If this particular activity were to be included in every American's daily exercise program, the need for knee and back surgery would be decreased and might even be eliminated. This is just one example of how muscular balance can protect a joint from stress and ultimately reduce skyrocketing medical costs.

Muscular balance also affects our posture. Proper posture does not mean the "stiff shoulders pulled back, stomach in, tense neck, toes turned out" military stance. Instead, a vertical profile plumb line should be seen to pass from the ear through the shoulder, elbow, hip, wrist, and ankle joints. Take a moment to stand in front of a mirror in profile view with your heels together and toes open in a tripod base. Notice how the weight sways forward out of the vertical line with the hips, shoulders, and head over the toes. Since muscles work in pairs, every pair will need to compensate for the displacement from the plumb (vertical) line. Thus, one half of the pair will work harder and become tighter. The other half will become weaker and over-stretched. Place your toes together. Separate your heels so the Achilles tendons are behind your third toes (center of your forefoot). Your body now has a more stable, rectangular base of support. Your body will sway back over your foot center, with your hips, shoulders, and head ideally aligned.

We all have within us the capacity to stand with correct posture. However, this capacity cannot be realized without proper training. Children model the behavior of their parents and other adults. It has recently been found that as early as forty-two minutes after birth, a newborn can imitate his mother's facial expression.

One day, when I was walking in a park with my daughter, who was five years old, she looked at my feet and how I was walking. She was walking with her feet pointing forward, but when she noticed my feet were turned outward, she turned her feet outward. After walking a few more steps, I turned my feet forward, and she turned her feet forward. I tested this several times, and she copied my way of walking each time. Children mimic what they see. Consequently, the incorrect use of the body may be handed down from one generation to another.

Ideally, principles of correct posture should begin in the developing years. But it is never too late to begin, and amazing changes can occur at any age. Dailey Inner Core Workout, based on Dr. Amy Cochran's Physio-Synthesis, is successful in correcting muscular imbalance and developing balanced alignment. The system applies the laws of physics to the body by developing the intrinsic, or core, muscles of the body. It will appeal to most exercise enthusiasts who are after a well-defined body, since the contour of the body and support of the spine and pelvis are dependent upon the intrinsic muscles.

The Dailey Inner Core Workout retrains muscle pairs to develop the weak half of the pair and relax the overdeveloped and often chronically tense half. Reeducation begins with the feet, the foundation of the body structure. In so doing, awareness is developed in the relationship between muscles that are not anatomically connected. Just as in "referred pain," the cause of neck, shoulder, and jaw pain may originate in the alignment of the feet or pelvis.

A unique feature of the Dailey Inner Core Workout is the development of a kinesthetic sense. Sometimes referred to as the "intelligence of the body," this sense allows individuals to feel the position and movement of their body parts. Reaction time and agility are affected by the transmission of information from their body parts to their brains by way of proprioceptors (the body's Global Positioning System, or GPS) *(fig. 10)*.

Proprioceptors are sense receptors located within every muscle, tendon, and joint. Proprioceptors and the vestibular apparatus, the body's balance sensor inside the inner ear, send messages to the brain. The inner ear contains fluid crystals and very small hair/nerve cell balance sensors. When the head leans forward, backward, or rotates around in circles, the fluid moves the crystals and hair cells; along with the proprioceptors, balance information is sent to the

FIGURE 10

inner ear balance sensors

Otoliths create movements in the glutinous layer that push the hair cells in the ear, helping us know our current positioning of the body and achieve our sense of balance.

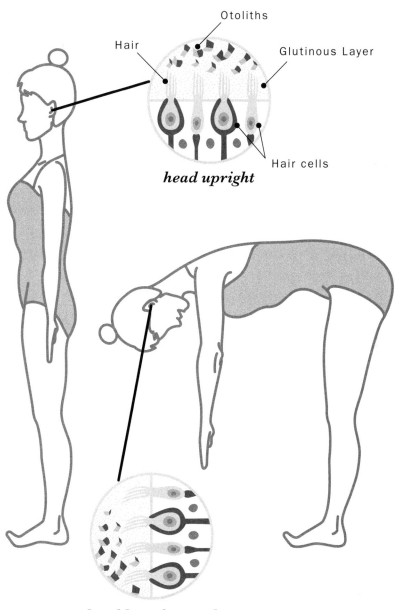

Otoliths

Hair

Glutinous Layer

Hair cells

head upright

head bent forward

brain. The brain then informs the body on how to stand up against gravity. A vertical plumb-line posture, along with balance and coordinated movements, is impossible without good proprioception and a well-balanced vestibular system. Imagine the proprioception capabilities of gymnasts!

If you have had poor posture for a long period of time, that posture will feel correct and straight to you. Your proprioceptors and vestibular system will have adapted to the misalignment. Then, should you stand in a vertical plumb line, there will be a feeling of leaning forward or backward, depending on your specific postural distortion. The Dailey Inner Core Workout is unique in that its movements will recalibrate your proprioceptors and vestibular apparatus and correct posture will begin to feel straight.

Time spent being physically active will have limited fitness benefits of strength training and aerobic activities without detailed information on balanced healthy body alignment and how our body compares to balanced alignment.

Overall Physical Fitness

The concept of physical fitness has broadened in recent years. Once defined according to cardiovascular function, according to the American College of Sports Medicine, fitness now also includes flexibility, agility, muscular strength, and body composition. Correct posture is essential for optimal body function and health, as well as for the body's shape to reach its potential. The Dailey Inner Core Workout gives people of all ages the tools to balance their muscle pairs and properly align themselves from head to toe. It improves our most common movements of standing, sitting, and walking and propels every athletic endeavor past our self-induced injuries. The fundamentals of the Dailey Inner Core Workout underline the fact that the best defense against injuries is a good offense using proper alignment and muscular balance.

In the words of my mentor and amazing Master Pilates teacher, Ron Fletcher, who wrote the book *Every Body is Beautiful:*

> Every body is divinely inspired, superbly designed, awesome in the complex way it's put together and wonderful in the simple, economical way it works. Every body can be vital, strong and flexible, moving through life with grace and assurance, totally healthy—not just some of the time but most of the time. Every body can be improved, inside and outside, because the body potential is hardly ever realized.

He also used the saying "at the ready" to describe the importance of flexibility and strength of unlocked joints in order to be ready for immediate corrective actions required to prevent an injury.

A beautiful, balanced physique is achieved through the support and balance of our deepest layers of muscles. There are four to six layers of muscles in all areas of our bodies. However, mainstream fitness facilities stress the importance of the superficial muscles, only giving minimal consideration to helping us achieve correct postural alignment, not realizing how it affects the quality of our lives, both physical and mental.

Muscle pairs work as the yin and yang of body transformation. When the intrinsic muscles are strengthened, shaped, and balanced, the outer, superficial muscles conform. This produces the ideal shape that nature intended. When our bodies achieve correct alignment due to this core muscle support, we move easily—requiring minimum effort for maximum results.

The Dailey Inner Core Workout trains us to balance muscle pairs from the inside out, using our minds every bit as much as our bodies. This joining of forces produces amazing changes in our body's shape and function. The method involves the technique of the physiologic "coming together" on all levels—physical, mental, and emotional. From this coming together, students make real improvements in the shape of their bodies and feel wonderful at the same time.

The first step is to neutralize (or clear) the mind and relax. Most of the movements take place on a mat so that the superficial muscles aren't activated by working against gravity. When lying supine (on your back with your face up), gravity helps us create a "plumb line" posture, broadening and opening our shoulders, flattening our abdominals, and balancing our head above our shoulders rather than in front of them, which is what often occurs when we stand.

The next step is to create new, balanced movement patterns. Each of us has numerous already-established and, most often, incorrect movement patterns. If we are unhappy with our body shape or the way it functions, this is due to dysfunctional patterns of our muscle pairs. Our body becomes a slave to this dysfunction because what it has previously learned prevents us from being able to perform a new movement correctly. We must first "unlearn" the previous pattern and then teach our body the new one.

Since old movement patterns will take over when executing fast or complex movements, the Dailey Inner Core Workout uses very slow, smooth movements with a feeling of gliding, sliding, or floating. The slow pace allows you to visualize while you are executing the movement and get a better feeling and understanding of the movement. This way the new neurological pattern is programmed into your nervous system without interference from your old pattern. The most notable aspect of our nervous system is its elasticity (its ability to change). Fortunately, the synaptic connections, the interconnections between nerves, can be changed at any time during our lives. The purpose of the Dailey method is to allow you to efficiently and effectively make the necessary changes in your movement patterns.

The Dailey Inner Core Workout also helps regulate your body weight by burning more calories from increased muscle mass in all layers of newly strengthened muscles, including your inner core. This workout also gives you two additional benefits: ideal body shape and mechanical function.

Growing older can also take a toll on our bodies if we don't take care of them. Many of the so-called "natural" effects of the aging process come about as a result of ignoring our injuries and chronic aches and pains until our body becomes deformed. For many of us, taking care of our bodies is not a priority, and thus some injuries are ignored and never completely heal. This causes adaptations in our nervous system, which brings about muscle changes, leading to deformities. This dysfunctional neuromuscular condition is the only logical explanation for how a perfectly shaped and functioning body at the age of five ends up twisted, bent, and distorted in old age. Prevention of such an unnecessary physical distortion can be achieved through participating regularly in a balanced, focused, and effective fitness program.

The increasing emphasis on the benefits of mind-body conditioning is evidenced by articles appearing in many national magazines, including *Shape, Self, Elle, Vogue, Glamour,* and *Mirabella*. The Dailey Inner Core Workout is the most effective, medically based, and interesting time-efficient method of fitness for the new millennium. Having your mind and body united and focused on practicing movements that retrain unbalanced muscle groups will allow the body to regain its natural balanced alignment.

Your health is your longest-held and most precious asset. It's with you from your first breath—you, like most babies, were probably born with good health. From day one, a baby's true and natural inclination is to make small, simple,

65

natural movements. Joint by joint they begin to move and make many repetitions, beginning with their mouth, eyes, fingers, and toes, then progressing on to wrists, elbows, and shoulders, knees, hips, and pelvis, and up the spine to the head and neck. Gradually, babies instinctively learn to roll over, sit up, crawl, stand, walk, jump, and run. This progressive movement is a natural learning experience.

If we continue to move as we did when we were children, we will still have the freely moving body and maintain the embryonic curve we were born with. Body maintenance is essential to have a natural, organic body to lead us through our life's journey. In some eastern countries, such as Japan, most citizens do not change their diet and the way they walk, stand, and sit as they age. They have not adopted the western ways of sitting in chairs and unhealthy eating habits.

Many of the physical problems we experience as we age are a result of a lack of body awareness plus a lack of information and education on how to efficiently use our body structure. Without a natural, "trued-up" body alignment, our six-hundred-plus muscles begin to weaken or tighten, pulling bones into an unnatural alignment that affects all systems of the body, including the respiratory, musculoskeletal, circulatory, nervous, organ, and glandular systems.

According to the book *Dare to Be 100* by geriatric expert Dr. Walter Bortz ll, the biggest predictor of whether a person will end up in a nursing home is the strength of the legs, not the strength of the heart. Your legs can make your heart stronger, but your heart can never make your legs stronger. Rather than an inevitable consequence of aging, the increased loss of muscle tissue as people get older is recognized more as the result of "use it or lose it," a sedentary death syndrome.

Just as the brain receives information from the eyes when the eyes are open, the brain receives GPS signals from proprioceptors in joints, tendons, and muscles when they are active. The brain, master of control, knows when your muscles are active and when they are inactive. It can detect the exact muscles that are not being used. If a muscle is not used for two days, on the third day, a 1 percent loss of muscle strength begins for each consecutive day it is not used. If inactive for thirty days, a 28 percent loss of muscle strength will occur. Each of our six hundred-plus muscles has a purpose. All of our muscles multitask, except for the diaphragm. Respiration is its sole purpose. When muscles atrophy, other muscles must fill in, putting more of a burden and stress upon them than is normal. Eventually, a problem will occur. The professional dance community has a saying: "If you miss one day of dance technique practice, you know it; if you miss two days, your teacher knows it; if you miss three days, the audience knows it . . . and you will lose your job."

Meditation 101

Mainstream medicine is finding that even brief stints of sitting quietly and thinking about your breath can improve concentration, lower stress, and perhaps reduce the risk of disease. In a study from the University of North Carolina, people who meditated for twenty minutes a day performed ten times better than their non-meditating peers on a test that measured focus (Listful).

The original purpose of the creation of yoga was a preparation to sit comfortably during meditation. A practice dating back thousands of years that has a strong spiritual component, it is now labeled a mind-body exercise method. Even thousands of years ago, there was a need for balance between physical flexibility and strength.

Traditional hatha yoga features a series of static poses along with breathing techniques and meditation with an emphasis on inward focus. With continued practice, one should be able to sit with ease in the crossed-leg position in order to meditate in comfort for twenty minutes. As many who have experienced this sitting position find, at first it may be uncomfortable or impossible.

Anyone who tries to sit still for a few seconds knows that the mind tends to jump around like a monkey. It naturally wanders to entertain one thought or another. In the practice of Zen meditation, the goal is to put a stop to this normal activity of the mind and let the restless mind come to a point of stillness.

Breath counting is one effective way of regulating our thoughts to enable the mind to focus on the here and now. How, then, do we deal with stray thoughts? The most effective way is to, each time you notice the mind has gone astray, recognize the stray thoughts as such and go back to breathing. An effective way to deal with stray thoughts is the way a mountain deals with clouds. The mountain is affected in no way at all by passing clouds but simply remains there, unmoved and unperturbed.

In Transcendental Meditation, another form of eastern meditation, a mantra is employed to help the practitioner focus the mind on one point. This is a word or short phrase given by the guru or meditation master to the practitioner, who then is invited to repeat the mantra with the breathing process during meditation. Devoting your attention to the mantra in this way mitigates the entry of irrelevant or stray thoughts and keeps the mind on a point of focus.

Some Christian spiritual directors have been adapting the use of the mantra for those they direct in meditation or contemplation, making use of a holy name or phrase from sacred scriptures that strikes a resonating chord in the practitioner. No matter the spiritual origin, the use of a mantra can be an effective way of quieting the mind to a point of focus.

Dr. Om Prakash, author of *From Change to Transformation & Beyond,* says the practice of meditation is the key to resting an overworked and never-ceasing mind. It balances the right brain, associated with emotion and creativity, with the left brain, associated with logic and reason. "In this culture the left brain—where there's constant chatter—is dominant. The right side just sits there like a bum. Meditation lets the left and right brain work together as one unit."

Meditation also restores equilibrium to crucial brain chemicals, serotonin, and dopamine. Serotonin regulates your mood and is responsible for feelings of pleasure and relaxation. (Low levels can trigger carbohydrate cravings.) Dopamine causes feelings of pleasure and helps you to maintain good functions, such as concentration.

To prepare for meditation Dr. Prakash says, "Close your eyes and be aware of your breath. Don't focus on your breath, just be aware of it." He explains that the difference between focus and awareness is akin to staring intently at a lamp versus simply knowing it's there, which takes less effort. He continues, "Breath is life. Breath controls the mind; the mind controls the body." Prakash says if you find yourself in a swirling tunnel of thought, don't resist or try to stop the thoughts; just notice them and let them pass.

Giving rest time to our overworked and never-ceasing mind is a life-sustaining routine. Albert Einstein said he got his best ideas when he went for a walk or ate an apple.

Regular participation in physical exercise, spiritual practice, family activities, and meditation will often make us more productive than spending extra hours at the office. In addition, when information is crowded into our brains without time for synthesis, we may as well not have received it at all. Research has shown that when information is taken in without regular breaks, very little is retained. When the same information is studied with regularly spaced breaks, recall performance is significantly higher. Time is needed for information to become knowledge. Even after elementary school, recess is still very important.

The maintenance of good mental health is hard work. Maintaining a meditation schedule of twenty minutes in the morning and twenty minutes in the evening, keeping your word, and honoring yourself are difficult tasks. The evening meditation could be active, as in a quiet walk. Never feel guilty about taking care of yourself. No one else can do it for you.

Another benefit for meditation may include weight loss. If you have an overworked mind, you may be experiencing stress. Your adrenal gland may be overworked and exhausted. The thyroid gland, which provides backup work for the adrenals, regulates the body's metabolism. If it is constantly covering work for the adrenals, its metabolic function will be weakened. After twenty years of failing to lose seventeen pounds, I began to meditate. Within a year, I had lost ten pounds. I believe the meditation brought my adrenal and thyroid glands back to a normal function. I'm much more relaxed, ideas come to me out of the blue, and I'm still a work in progress, practicing meditation and also losing weight.

Kinesthetic Awareness

Developing a kinesthetic sense of your body, a self-observation of knowing where your body parts are and how they are moving, is essential to gain and maintain corrective changes from physical movement instruction. Imagine the details an artist can *see* when looking at texture and shades of light to reproduce a scene on canvas. Imagine the details a musician can *hear* when listening to the rhythms and intervals of sound during a musical performance. Dance performers must mentally connect and *feel* their whole body in order to express their story through movement.

Just as an artist must see and a musician must hear and a dancer must feel the movements, the Dailey Inner Core Workout method leads you to feel your body. You will learn how to move in a way never felt before and build a virtuo-so level of body awareness through refined movement. You must also listen to the Dailey Inner Core Workout video instructor and visually notice how your body is moving during the movements. All three sensory systems are important in the learning journey. The process of developing a heightened sense of body awareness is an important element in creating an aesthetic body. Every body has the facility to become uniquely beautiful when brought to its potential. The method guides you to develop an attractive body that functions with ease and efficiency without aches and pains.

The majority of Americans live their lives in a dissociated state—mind and body are treated as separate entities. A common fitness regimen is exercising on a treadmill or stationary bicycle while watching TV or listening to vocal music. In the past, conventional physical fitness and medical treatment models fostered this belief, rarely linking the status of one to the other. This belief system has resulted in a status quo in which individuals depend upon external forces to "fix" their bodies or minds, unaware of their own innate ability to attain and sustain a mind-body fitness balance. The Dailey Inner Core Workout is a unique method of interconnectedness between mind and body to achieve holistic fitness, emphasizing the empowerment of the individual to be aware of their body, the need for fitness, and the knowledge to make the appropriate life changes to achieve it. The method is mentally as well as physically challenging. One of my students said it well, "Aerobics was boring. This method stimulated me intellectually. Before I took these classes, I was just a disconnected set of parts."

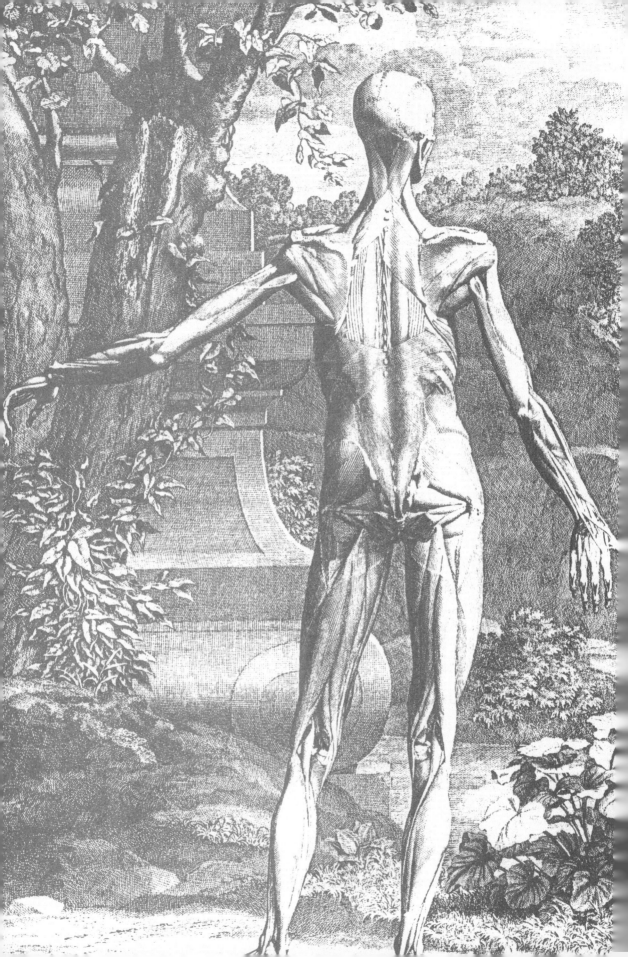

PART TWO

THE WAY IT WORKS

"I HEAR, AND I FORGET. I SEE, AND I REMEMBER. I DO, AND I UNDERSTAND."

—CHINESE PROVERB

DAILEY INNER CORE WORKOUT

Let's move now to options on how to stay healthy and prevent numerous physical ailments. The Dailey Inner Core Workout is about to begin. The late 1800s to early 1900s was a time when innovative methods for physical fitness were created by Amy Cochran, MD, DO (1882–1961), Joseph Pilates (1883–1967), Matthias Alexander (1869–1955), and Moshe Feldenkrais (1904–1984). Reeducation through their methods provides a process to transform a person's unbalanced postural alignment into its natural, healthy, organic alignment and function.

We will be working in standing, supine, and prone positions while doing the Dailey Inner Core Workout. Keep in mind that when the body is healthy and balanced, all body parts directly and indirectly create a physical synthesis through all of their connections between the feet and head. You will know your mind and your body have found the connections when you feel a sensation of muscle action at the cranium (above the eyebrows, across the bridge of your nose, and behind your ears) when you move your toes and ankles.

Two vertical lines will give you a visual image of ideal structural body alignment. From a profile view, the vertical line will pass from your head, centered above your shoulders in a neutral, balanced alignment with a normal curve at the neck and the opening of your ear in a vertical position. With your shoulders broad, the profile vertical line continues to pass down through the center of your shoulder joints, elbows, hips, wrists, knees, and ankles *(fig. 11)*.

With your pelvis in balanced (neutral) alignment, your symphysis pubis (pubic bone) and anterior superior iliac spine (ASIS/hip points) are in the same vertical line. Your ischial tuberosities (sit bones) reach toward your heels. This places your pelvis and hips in balanced alignment, neither extended rooster tail nor flexed sad-dog tail. Your knee joints (neither flexed or hyperextended) will point forward, with your ankle joints ready for movement, and your legs will be vertical at a right angle to your feet. Your hips, knees, and ankles, in a neutral position, are "at the ready" for movement and are able to function as shock absorbers, providing a cushion for pressure on your joints as every step is taken. This alpha posture will allow unblocked, free-flowing blood circulation.

The front (anterior) vertical midline passes between your eyes, the center of your nose, chin, sternum (breastbone), navel, pubic bone, and where your knees and big toes come together. Your inner ankles are very close to the vertical line.

Six horizontal lines have a balanced relationship with the two vertical lines. Horizontal lines include the lines between your eyes, ears, shoulders, hips, knees, and ankles. Due to our habitual right- or left-handed movements, one shoulder, hip, eye, or ear may be higher than its opposite partner. This creates an imbalance of muscle partners between your shoulders and head and of partners between your hips and low ribs. When your body has balanced muscle partners, all horizontal lines will be level.

FIGURE 11

vertical line posture

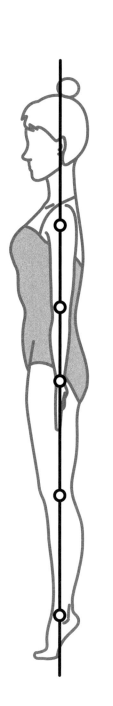
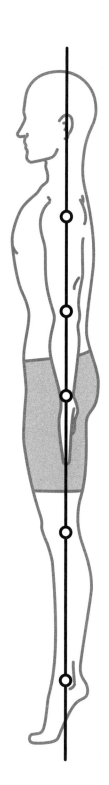

In order for us to understand how areas of our body interact, we must be aware of the body's structure of musculature and ligaments. Our hips have six layers of muscles. Other areas have four to five layers. The surface layer muscles are large. As muscle layers progress to the core, muscle fibers decrease in size and length. The shortest muscle fibers are found around our joints. These inner core muscles, along with the ligaments that lie beneath them, are essential to stabilize our joints. Every muscle layer must have the same quality of muscle strength, even though they vary in length.

Each muscle has a partner, and their function is the opposite of each other, such as flexion (bending at a joint) versus extension (opening at a joint). When they are balanced in their strength and united in action, they are able to provide the activated, continuous joint stability that is necessary for maintaining erect posture and offsetting the pull of gravity.

The goal of the Dailey Inner Core Workout in developing erect posture is to balance the body from bottom to top, front to backside, and right side to left side so that all movements spiral upward, allowing the body to express the positive half of the law of gravitation. The body will be able to maintain its erectness and perform its function without the rigidity of surface muscles. In this way, gravity can positively influence erect posture. I had a lesson in 1998 with Dr. Lucille Coughran, one of the first Physio-Synthesis teachers, who was trained by Dr. Amy Cochran. Dr. Lucille told us that the destructive forces exerted by rigidity of structure are exemplified by the type of large buildings that existed prior to earthquake laws. At that time, multi-storied buildings were not constructed with materials that allowed for sway.

Considering the number of segments in the body and the oscillating movement that is normal, fitness practices that focus on the development of the outer muscles to the exclusion of inner core muscles should be viewed warily. If you have rigid surface muscles, they will lock out the core muscles that allow the body to sway and prevent the body from being at the ready. The old saying "It is not the walls but the supporting structure that holds up a building" also holds true in the Dailey Inner Core Workout.

Your body has a unique design concept for maintaining erect posture. The concept revolves around six interrelated areas that make up the core supportive structure of your body. Each serves as a critical area of support and can be graphically represented by a triangular design. Triangles are not absolute structures and may vary from one person to another. They serve as a visual technique for illustrating points of support, proper weight distribution, and the "narrowing" principle.

When your muscles are balanced with all straight vertical and horizontal lines, you will be able to assume the following four positions due to performing regular maintenance of your true, natural original body. Try these four activities and evaluate whether you can do each of them:

> Squat down and sit with your feet flat on the floor and your sit bones near your heels.

> Sit on the floor with your knees together pointing forward and your hips sitting on your heels with your feet pointing backward away from your knees.

> Stay in the above position with your knees slightly apart. Place your head on the floor as your hips rest on your heels. This is the child pose, the embryonic curve position in which we developed when we were in our mothers' wombs.

> Kneel as do Japanese women wearing a kimono — knees on the floor, toes "on the walk," heels lifted, and hips on your heels.

How did you perform? Were these easy? If not, you need a plan to accomplish them.

Many people can relate to the importance of maintaining their car. Cars run best and avoid breakdowns when they are regularly maintained. They also begin to lose value the minute you drive them off the lot. Compare your body to an automobile. You can help reverse depreciation of your most valuable possession (your body) with a regular tune-up. You cannot trade in your body for a new one as you can a car. The Dailey Inner Core Workout, practiced two to four times weekly, will provide your body with a regular tune-up and accomplish the following: rear-end alignment; joint lubrication; balanced "wheels" and "tire alignment"; spare tire removal; reconditioned frame; tension adjustment; hip and shoulder rotation; spinal alignment; shock absorber maintenance; and depreciation reversal.

The Dailey Inner Core Workout Triangles will provide you a complete safety inspection and help you design the maintenance program that is best for you.

Triangles

To begin, the maintenance program must start with the true structural foundation required for balanced posture. There are six triangles (*fig. 12*), which include your ankles, knees, hips, lower back, shoulders, eyes, and ears. The triangles are connected to the vertical lines, and your body must maintain the vertical and horizontal connections during the movements in order to maintain a healthy body function. All of your body parts—muscles, tendons, ligaments, organs, glands, nerves, arteries, and veins—are affected by the alignment of your body. If balanced alignment is not maintained, your energy (chi) will not flow through to all parts of your body. Compare the circulation of your body energy to an e-mail. If one letter or symbol is missing on your recipient's e-mail address, your message will not go through (*figs. 13 & 14*).

TRIANGLE 1

Apex: Ankle joints.

Base Line: Left to right inner heel of foot.

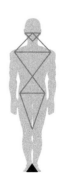

Position Options: Sit or lie on a mat in supine position with your feet placed the same as standing in flexed position and at a right angle to your lower leg to eliminate the effects of staying erect in the force of gravity. The feet can also be in the plantar-flexed (pointed) position *(fig. 15)*.

Lie on a mat in prone position with your feet plantar-flexed, big toes and toe joints together, little toes and outer border of feet on mat, heels apart with ankles tilted inward.

A structure is only as strong as its foundation, and you need to use the correct placement to provide the best foundation. When all triangles are in alignment, your body will be prepared for any challenge, due to its strength, agility, and oscillating movement. You will be able to feel muscle action from your feet through to your head.

In standing position, place your feet parallel at a right angle to your legs and face forward with your big toes together and your heels separated by approximately the width of three fingers. This will shift weight from your little toe metatarsals toward the first, second, and third metatarsals (ball of foot bones) that attach to your toes, giving you stronger structural support. The parallel foot position aligns the third toes, center of the forefoot, with the center of the heels and Achilles tendons. Your feet should tilt inward, placing your ankles close to the anterior mid-vertical line and lifting the outer border (arch) of your feet as your heels retain their distance apart. Notice that your knees turn inward as your ankles reach toward your midline. This issue will be addressed by Triangle 2—narrowed hips—and Triangle 3—lengthened lower back lumbar spine.

FIGURE 12

six structural triangles

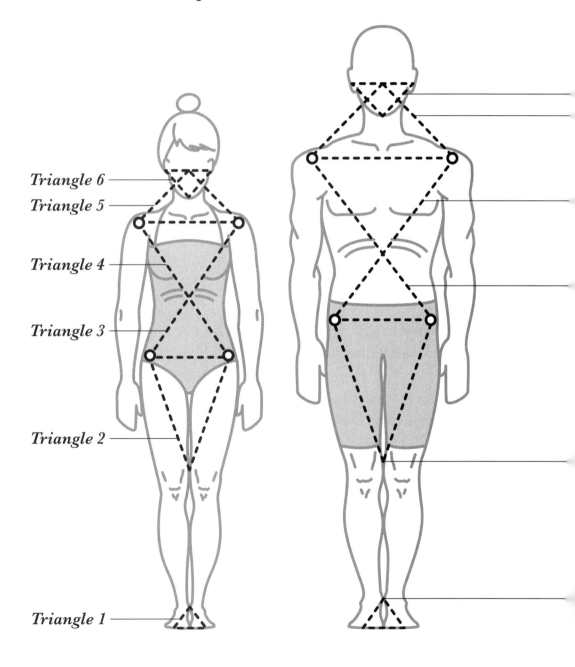

Triangle 6

Triangle 5

Triangle 4

Triangle 3

Triangle 2

Triangle 1

▲ 6

APEX: central portion of Mandible (lower jaw bone, chin)
BASE LINE: left to right Temporomandibular joint (TMJ)
near opening of your ear with Apex of Triangle 5 centered
over the Base Line of Triangle 6.

▲ 5

APEX: joint between the skull and atlas C1
cervical (neck) vertebra
BASE LINE: left to right shoulder

▲ 4

APEX: L1 & T12 connecting point
BASE LINE: left to right shoulder

▲ 3

APEX: Connecting point of the L1 lumbar & T12
thoracic vertebrae behind low end of the sternum
BASE LINE: Left to right hip with the addition
of the pelvis & sacrum

▲ 2

APEX: inner knee joints
BASE LINE: left to right hip

▲ 1

APEX: ankle joints
BASE LINE: left to right inner heel of foot

FIGURE 13
balanced & unbalanced knees

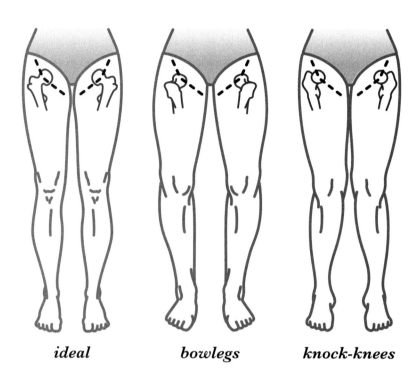

ideal   *bowlegs*   *knock-knees*

FIGURE 14
foot alignment

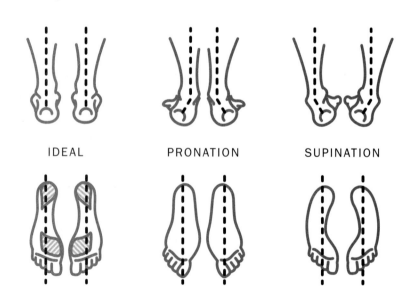

IDEAL   PRONATION   SUPINATION

Triangle 1 Benefits: Slenderizes your feet and ankles with strong muscular support for the four arches of your feet; allows for flexible unlocked ankles at the ready to absorb shock from movement; reshapes your inner and outer calf muscles; strengthens your inner thigh, core gluteal, and lower abdominal muscles; allows your toes and feet to function as a "second heart"; narrows your hips; creates the "walk the line" gait of fast-running athletes and fashion models.

A strong communication exists between your vestibular apparatus (the hearing and body position sensor of the inner ear) and proprioceptors at every joint, tendon, and muscle of your feet. With twenty-six bones in your feet, you have many proprioceptors that send information to your brain and improve balance. If your feet are rigid and not properly aligned, your brain will receive a minimum amount of information; this is similar to closing your eyes while you're trying to see what's in front of you.

Many children naturally have Triangle 1 foot alignment—that is, until they begin to copy their adult role models, who have lost their natural stance. They also have good balance sense from fun opportunities that develop their sense of balance, such as swinging, spinning, and turning upside down on monkey bars. Perhaps we should continue to play at playgrounds as adults, also!

Triangle 1 Prevents: Bunions; hammer toes; tender feet; swelling in the feet, ankles, and forelegs; waddle walk gait; migraine headaches; motion sickness; broad hips; mushy buttocks; toenail fungus; and callus under the little toe metatarsals. Narrow hips are impossible without parallel foot alignment and weight away from the little toe metatarsals.

When I was twenty-one, I developed bunions in my feet. The podiatrist advised me to stop wearing my fashionable, pointed-toe shoes and switch to lace-up shoes. I also learned that when walking with the knees and feet turned outward,

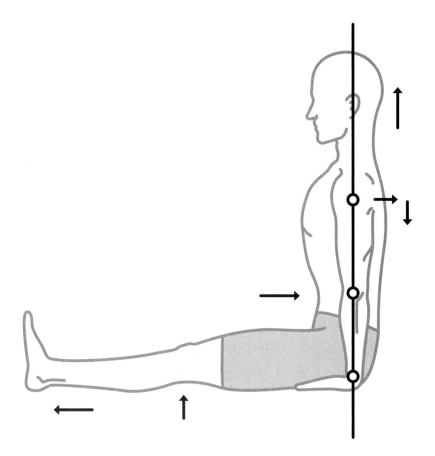

FIGURE 15

sitting: legs extended & supine

*Only if you turn your elbows outward are you activating your
muscles at the shoulder and back of the neck.*

the big toe is the last part of your foot to be anchored on the ground, causing a major possibility of bunion development. The opposite happens with the feet in Triangle 1 position. When the toes are inward, they are the first part of your foot to be anchored and are in their natural, balanced alignment.

One of my students who carried his weight on the outer part of his foot had a huge callus on the soles of his feet. It covered half of the sole of each foot from the middle (third) toe and center of the heel to the outer edge! He eventually had to have knee surgery due to his unbalanced stance.

Another student I worked with suffered from migraine headaches that began when she was in high school. Her doctor's solution was to give her medications. Her headaches continued into her late thirties, until she began to take Dailey Inner Core Workout classes. She had extremely tight muscles in her feet, which caused the muscles of her head to tighten, preventing the sacro-occipital (low spine sacrum to head) pump action *(figs. 16–17)*. Tight head muscles were giving her the headaches. After a month of classes with a focus on Triangle 1 and gradually gaining more flexibility and movement in her feet and ankles, her headaches went away.

TRIANGLE 2

Apex: Inner Knee Joints.

Base Line: Left to right hip.

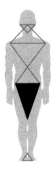

Position Options: Lie on a mat in supine position. Place your knees together, soft and unlocked with a reaching action toward the feet, assisting your hips to narrow and your lumbar spine to lengthen.

Maintain Triangle 1 to provide you a strong foundation. Feel the core muscles that surround your knee joints when they are unlocked and together on the vertical midline. Roll

FIGURE 16
cranial motion on inhalation and exhalation

inhalation

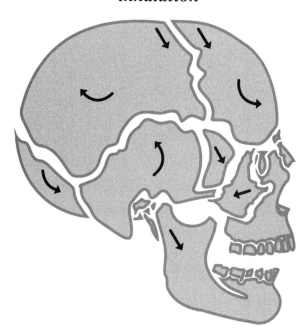

exhalation

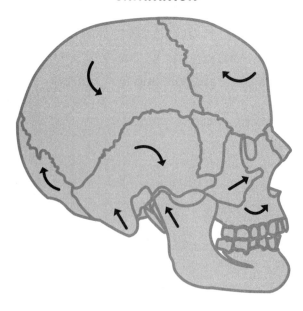

your hip points back, the pubic bone upward, and sit bones down toward your heels to lengthen the back of your waist (lumbar spine) and front of your hips (iliopsoas muscle). The purpose of the iliopsoas muscle, which is connected to the five lumbar vertebrae and the thigh bone, is flexion of the hip joint. If it is too tight, the inability to lengthen the front of your hip and lumbar spine will make it extremely difficult to place your pelvis in neutral and narrow your hips.

When your lumbar spine is lengthened, your hips will narrow and your knees will point forward, placing the femurs (thigh bones) into the ideal alignment at the hip sockets. A hollow space will appear below your anterior ribs with your core abdominals at work and your surface abdominals in natural rather than six-pack, armored mode. Your inner thighs will be together except for two small spaces—one above your knees and a small space below the pubic bone. In order to reap the benefits of Triangle 2, which include circulation and chi energy, you must maintain Triangle 1.

The Triangle 2 base from hip to hip is the foundation for the low-back lumbosacral spine and has a major part in strengthening the pelvic floor muscles. I saw how well this works several years ago with one of my students. She had pelvic girdle muscles that were weakened and stressed after having five children. She struggled with incontinence when she coughed, laughed, and sneezed. She had been taking Pilates classes, but when she added Inner Core Workout classes to her schedule, she was pleasantly surprised that her bladder issues subsided.

The Triangle 2 base line is horizontal from hip to hip. The head of the femur (thigh bone) fits better into the hip socket when the femur is flexed at a ninety degree angle to the trunk, as in a crawl position. This position places the femur heads in a horizontal position at the hips with the knees pointing forward and provides a balanced distribution of pressure on

FIGURE 17

occipital pump on inhalation and exhalation

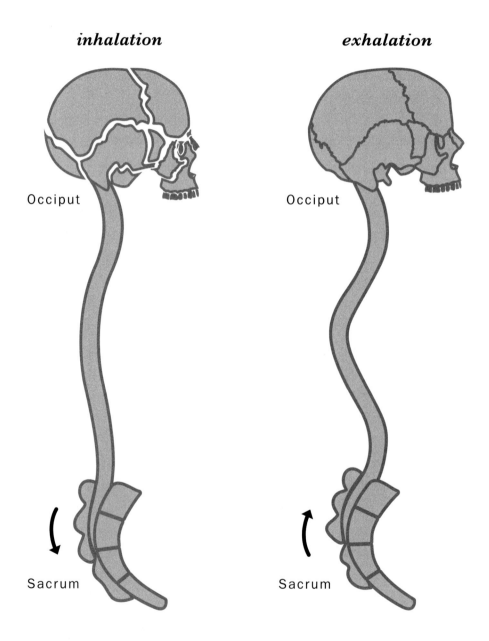

inhalation *exhalation*

Occiput Occiput

Sacrum Sacrum

the menisci, tendons, and ligaments of the femur knee joint and patella (knee cap). Triangle 2 allows the body to maintain the crawl position benefits to the hips and knees when taking the body to standing.

Often, people are not aware of Triangle 2 and its importance in maintaining health. If your inner knees are not together with knee caps facing forward and your knees are hyperextended, the possibility of developing avascular necrosis/osteonecrosis (death of the bones) at your hip and knee joints increases. Many people, especially women, hyperextend (lock) their knees, creating an imbalance of core and surface muscle partners that blocks circulation to the bones of the knee joints, dries up synovial (lubricating) fluid, and eventually results in the death of bone tissue due to a lack of blood supply. It can lead to tiny breaks in the bone and the eventual collapse of the bone, leading to knee replacement. Necrosis is primarily found in joints at the shoulders, knees, and hips, with hip joints most commonly affected.

I became aware of limited circulation to my knee joints one spring when I began wearing shorts. For a period of time, I sat in a squat position and then changed to sitting with my legs extended. My knees turned red from increased blood flow and stayed red for an hour! I got the message. Locking my knees was a habit I had to change. I also had to change my habit of standing and walking with my knees and feet turned outward, which also placed pressure on the medial side of my knee joint and was progressing into pain.

Another benefit of rebuilding stability in my hyperextended knees was the disappearance of the SI (sacroiliac) joint pain I had experienced for seventeen years. The pain began after the birth of my daughter. No treatments, physical therapy, chiropractic, or osteopathic helped. I eventually learned that when giving birth, the hormone relaxin is released to facilitate the birthing process by relaxing pelvic girdle musculature. I realized my hyperextended knees also caused the lateral hamstrings to overstretch, and their attachments to the sacrum and ilium were not able to secure the SI joints. With constant awareness and the desire to make changes, I now have healthy, pain-free knees and SI joints.

Triangle 2 Benefits: Corrects a shortened leg and dysfunction of hip joints; narrows hips; lengthens lumbar spine (back of waist); relaxes tense surface rectus-abdominals (abs, six-pack). Your inner core control takes over with the release of outer abdominal tension. Triangle 2 strengthens your quadriceps; activates your core abs, inner thighs, and pelvic floor muscles; develops toned gluteal muscles. Feel your gluteal muscles activate, lift, and smile.

Triangle 2 Prevents: Pain in the knees, hips, lower back, and sacroiliac; broad hips; bird legs; sagging gluteal and low abdominal muscles; urinary incontinence and prolapsed organs. No need for adult diapers.

TRIANGLE 3

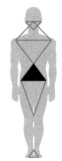

Apex: Connecting point of the L1 lumbar and T12 thoracic vertebrae behind low end of the sternum.

Base Line: Left to right hip with the addition of the pelvis and sacrum.

Position Options: Lie on a mat in supine position with the L1-T12 joint apex making an imprint into the mat and waistline rolled back to lengthen front of hips; place SI joint dimples against the mat and create a balanced lumbar curve, narrow hips, and core abdominal hollow below the front ribs.

Maintain Triangles 1 and 2. Lie on a mat in prone position, press pubic bone toward mat, and reach back of waist away from the mat to lengthen front of hips and lumbar curve, activate hip-narrowing and core abdominal muscles, and balance all pelvic girdle muscles to place it into neutral position.

The L1-T12 joint apex is essential to the maintenance of erect posture. It is the connecting point between the upper and lower torso. When back vertebral muscles are balanced, your back will be flat like a young child's back, without a trace of an indented spine between tense vertebral muscles. To position your pelvis in the neutral position described in Triangle 2, roll your hip points backward, your pubic bone upward, and your sit bones down toward your heels to lengthen the front of your hips and back of your waist, and narrow your hips. Broaden your lowest back ribs to activate your core abdominals and establish an anchoring point for the apex of Triangle 3 with a visual indicator of an abdominal hollow below your front ribs.

Triangle 3 Benefits: Strengthens your anterior core spinal muscles to balance with lengthened posterior spinal muscles; maintains alignment of vertebral bodies and arches; strengthens core and surface abdominal muscles; strengthens pelvic floor muscles; narrows hips; tones gluteal muscles; provides ideal space for pelvic girdle organs and glands; anchors the lumbar spine when performing footwork on the Pilates Reformer.

Triangle 3 Prevents: Pain in lumbar spine, hips, sacrum, knees, and possibility for arthritis in lower extremities; herniated spinal discs; broad hips; sagging abdominal and gluteal muscles; urinary incontinence; prolapsed organs. I learned of an extreme example of what could happen if we neglect to take care of our bodies from a neighbor. She was a single woman in her early 80s and was very computer savvy. She volunteered weekly at a charity organization's office and regularly took walks in her neighborhood. As a Christian Scientist, she did not go to a doctor until she had an extremely severe problem. Her bladder, uterus, and intestinal lining fell out of her pelvis almost midway to her knees. They would sling against her legs as she walked. She eventually went to a doctor, and the surgery to repair it was successful.

During a class, when I was teaching the importance of Triangle 3 and movements that build its muscle strength and support, I mentioned this example of what happened to my neighbor. After class, a student told me that when her husband was in medical school, he worked in the hospital emergency room, and a woman who had urinary incontinence came in for treatment. She had stuffed a potato into her body, like a tampon, to prevent her organs from falling out—and it had sprouted! She had to have surgery to solve the problem.

In both of these examples, the women could have prevented these extreme results by practicing correct Triangle 3 form. The management of Triangle 3 is extremely important to your overall health.

TRIANGLE 4

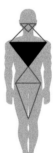

Apex: L1 and T12 connecting point.

Base Line: Left to right shoulder.

Position Options: Lie on a mat in supine position, and, as suggested by Master Pilates teacher Ron Fletcher, place your shoulder blades flat on the mat. Imagine wearing jeans, and "slide your shoulder blades down toward your back jean pockets," the top of your sternum toward the ceiling and your head, low end of sternum toward the mat and your feet.

In standing position, maintain Triangles 1, 2, and 3 to provide a stable foundation. Widen the clavicles (collarbones) to flatten the scapula (shoulder blades) against your back ribs. Keep your sternum vertical by reaching in opposition action like a bow and arrow, with the top of the sternum forward and up and the low end backward and down. Anchoring the lower sternum back and down is essential in order to stabilize the L1-T12 apex of Triangle 4, which is the same apex as Triangle 3. Feel how the muscle pairs work together.

To Triangle 4, add the connection of arms hanging in a profile, a vertical line running from the shoulders through the elbows, wrists, and hands. A straight medial line should run from the elbow through the wrist and middle finger. If the line is not straight and the hand turns outward, muscles will become tense through the shoulders to the neck and head. I learned this from another student who had migraine headaches. Her hands always turned outward. When I tested her hand position myself, I could immediately feel a great amount of tension in my cranial muscles. I was on my way to a headache, also.

Here is another example of the importance of the connection of the arms to Triangle 4. I was not aware that shoulder joints could develop avascular necrosis/osteonecrosis until a relative began to have extreme pain in his left shoulder joint. He worked as an engineer for a company that developed printing equipment and spent many of his hours as a draftsman. His left elbow and forearm would be resting on the draft board, and, while drawing with his right hand, he would lean on his left elbow. This compressed his humerus (upper bone of the arm from the elbow) into his left shoulder joint and blocked blood flow to the area. He eventually had to have surgery due to necrosis of the bones in his shoulder joint.

The next detail in achieving this proper form is extremely important for toned triceps and stable shoulder joints, provided by strong rotator cuff muscles. Turn your elbows outward to open space (elbow windows) for your ribs to expand. Feel the engaged and toned muscles of the triceps, latissimus dorsi (lats, love handles), core shoulder girdle, and low abdominal muscles when the elbows turn outward. If your shoulders are rounded, you will not be able to receive the feeling because the core muscle connection does not go through. To reap the benefits of practicing Dailey Inner Core Workout sessions, all triangles must be balanced and working together.

Triangle 4 Benefits: A broad shoulder frame allows space for the lungs to expand front to back, side to side, and up and down, providing efficient breathing and increased respiratory capacity; provides a stable base for the arms and shoulders to move easily with support; positions the head centered above the shoulders; allows balanced rotator cuff muscles and toned triceps.

Triangle 4 Prevents: Pain in shoulders and neck; forward head position; possibility for arthritis in upper extremities; rotator cuff problems; flabby triceps; flabby latissimus dorsi; dowager hump; thyroid problems; scoliosis; asthma and respiratory problems.

TRIANGLE 5

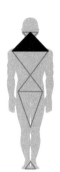

Apex: Joint between the skull and atlas C1 cervical (neck) vertebra.

Base Line: Left to right shoulder.

Position Options: Lie on a mat in supine position, your head centered with a balanced cervical curve, chin toward your breastbone, the backs of your ears and crown of your head reaching away from your shoulders, and the opening of the ear horizontal.

Lie on a mat in prone position, your forehead on the mat with your chin toward your breastbone, cervical spine reaching away from the mat.

Maintain Triangles 1, 2, 3, and 4. Lengthen and broaden Triangle 5 to support the shoulder girdle. Keep your head centered with a balanced cervical curve. If your shoulders are rounded forward, a balanced cervical curve will be impossible.

Triangle 5 Benefits: Lengthened cervical spine; oxygen reaching the brain; no wrinkled or green skin microbiome on folded wrinkle tissue from lack of oxygen at back of neck; support for shoulder girdle and skull; head correctly centered above the shoulders; improved vision; cranial micro movement; toned neck and facial muscles; broad shoulders; good balance; open nasal passages; oxygen reaching back of throat to prevent whitish sulfur-producing bacteria on the tongue, which causes bad breath and may join with food debris to form tonsil stones.

Triangle 5 Prevents: Pain in neck; motion sickness; balance problems; falls; laryngitis; congested nasal passages; wax build up in ear; swimmer's ear; dry eyes; hair loss; double chin; saggy front of neck, ear lobes, and facial muscles; wrinkled or green skin at back of neck; weight gain; receding gums; whitish tongue, bad breath, and tonsil stones.

People who are overweight tend to have heavy subluxations (dislocations) in the region of the upper first, second, third, and fourth cervical vertebrae. The lower fifth vertebra of the neck is pulled forward as well. This position of the vertebrae produces pressure on the nerves that prepare, appropriate, and consume nutriment, renovate the body, and keep it in normal form and functioning condition. A great quantity of extra fat and other chemical substances that are meant to be used by the nutriment system will pile up in the body.

The fatty substances are not being consumed and appropriated normally due to the abnormal placement of some of the vertebrae or ribs. This alignment interferes with the consumption of the fat and with production of the fuel that should have been produced by it. When undisturbed, the abdomen, heart, and lungs bring the food in for use. Because it is not used, the tissues store up an oversupply, causing a fat and flabby condition.

TRIANGLE 6

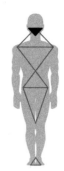

Apex: Central portion of mandible (lower jaw bone, chin).

Base Line: Left to right temporomandibular joint (TMJ) near the opening of your ear, with apex of Triangle 5 centered over the base line of Triangle 6.

Position Options: In standing position, to balance your neck curve, level your head, place the outer opening of your ears in a vertical line, and point your chin downward toward your sternum with the backs of your ears and crown of your head pointing upward away from your shoulders.

Lie on a mat in supine position with the opening of your ear horizontal and your head centered as in standing position.

Lie on a mat in prone position, your forehead on the mat with your chin toward your breastbone, your cervical spine reaching away from the mat.

Maintain Triangles 1 to 5. To place your head level and balanced over the pelvis and shoulder girdle, lower your chin toward your sternum and reach the backs of your ears away from your shoulders.

The vestibular apparatus, which is located within your inner ear, functions as the body's director of equilibrium. The fluid and tiny hair/nerve cells located within the semicircular canals of the inner ear are active in maintaining stability of the head and body when they are motionless. They also balance your head and body when they are suddenly moved or rotated. Positioning of the joints is detected by proprioceptors, located at every joint, tendon, and muscle. The brain's cerebellum is important in interpreting impulses from your inner ear. This information allows the nervous system to predict the consequences of rapid body movements. Your brain can then send motor impulses to stimulate appropriate skeletal muscles so that loss of balance may be prevented.

You'll know that your head is in its balanced, level position when the opening of your ear is vertical and your jaw hangs as in a sling from the Triangle 6 base line. Your teeth will not touch, and your head will slightly nod (like the way a horse's head moves) when you are walking.

Feel core and surface shoulder girdle muscles when your head is level. Feel your low abdominal, pelvic floor, and core abdominal hollow muscles engage when your head is level and Triangles 1 to 5 are balanced. Feel cranial (head) muscles lift the face above the brow line, broaden the bridge of the nose, open the nasal passages to allow oxygen to reach the back of your throat, and tighten the abdominal and gluteal muscles when the backs of your ears and crown of your head reach upward, away from the shoulders. A recent study by David Kahan and Robert Shaw reported that as facial muscles weaken, cranial bone density decreases and the shape of the face changes (Parker).

I learned how muscles can affect the shape of bones when I was in the fifth grade. I began to experience growing pains, and a lump below my kneecaps started to appear. My leg muscles couldn't keep up with the growing pace of my thigh bones, and I was having an Osgood-Schlatter experience.

During the teen years, a growth spurt causes repeated stress from contraction of the quadriceps through the patellar tendon to the immature tibial tuberosity at the knees. This can cause inflammation of the tendon, leading to excess bone growth in the tuberosity, which produces a visible lump. My lump is still visible today. Another example of excess bone growth happened in my forties. I began to have discomfort behind my right collarbone. At a chiropractic exam, the doctor said there was an issue with my thyroid gland, which is positioned near the collarbones. After his treatment, the pain went away, but the medial end of my right collarbone is still slightly larger than the left.

Triangle 6 Benefits: Releases facial tension; provides static and dynamic equilibrium; maintains strength of cranial muscles, cranial bone density, shape, and ageless appearance; opens nasal passages and allows oxygen into back of the throat.

Triangle 6 Prevents: Abnormal wrinkling of face; balance problems; falls; motion sickness; the need for a face lift; whitish, sulfur-producing bacteria on your tongue, bad breath, and tonsil stones; laryngitis.

Examples: Australian actor Matthias Alexander experienced chronic laryngitis when he performed. Doctors couldn't help him, so he searched for a solution on his own and discovered the cause. He began to notice that when performing, he would collect excess tension in his shoulders and neck. His shoulder alignment would change into a protective position with his shoulders forward and toward his ears, causing his head placement to be slightly forward with the chin lifted. He had not been aware that he had excess tension in his shoulders that put stress on his larynx, causing laryngitis. He began to find new ways to speak and move with greater ease, keeping the back of his neck long and shoulders broad and relaxed with his head level. He learned to keep his Triangle 6 balanced.

I learned about tonsil stones and their cause from my daughter when she researched to find information about the small white stones she discovered in her throat. When oxygen is not reaching the back of your throat, whitish, sulfur-producing bacteria will develop and appear on your tongue, causing bad breath. The combination of food debris with sulfur-producing bacteria will form tonsil stones. Having the placement of your "head on straight" has many benefits, and it is essential for maintenance of your overall health.

With all triangles and vertical lines working together to add length and strength to your body, you may regain inches of your height. I have had students who regularly attended a Dailey Inner Core Workout class regain inches they had lost. At least three students gained an additional three-fourths of an inch, making them taller than ever measured in their adult life! You may actually be able to increase your height and "add years to your life and life to your years."

INNER CORE WORKOUT STRUCTURAL BALANCE TRAINING

This chapter provides information on movements that reeducate areas of the body that have lost their true purpose and maintain those that are purpose-efficient. Every muscle has a partner, and they work together with other muscle partners. They must all be in a strong relationship with a balance between strength and flexibility to be able to function in unison and provide ease of movement in all activities. Their united strength is essential to lengthen the spine from both ends, as well as to anchor the ends to maintain the spine's lengthened condition, a benefit to all systems of the body.

All triangles are involved in every Dailey Inner Core Workout movement. While the task of one triangle may be movement, the other triangles stabilize their position in order for the whole body to receive muscle activity connections and benefits. When practicing Triangle 1 foot movements, it is essential that the placements of Triangles 2 to 6 are in their assigned positions for the whole body to benefit. Remember the e-mail analogy! Did it go through? Those who can feel the muscle connection all the way through to their head when their toes move will receive a whole-body workout.

The pace of movements must be slow. Many body parts will be included in the movement or in stabilization. If the pace is too fast, the brain will not receive all the details from the neuromuscular reeducation message in order to make the necessary changes. Imagine three people speaking to you at the same time. Would you be able to hear all the details each person was saying? How does your computer respond when you quickly type in the characters?

I heard a good example of the importance of slow movement during a church service. The minister, who also played piano, was a stage manager when he attended Texas A&M University. He was getting the stage ready when Vladimir Horowitz came to the concert hall to get a feel for the piano and prepare for the concert he was to perform. The stage manager was very excited; he would be able to hear him play some of his concert music.

Horowitz began practicing scales with the right hand at whole-note (four beats) tempo up and down all eighty-eight keys. He played the same format with the left hand and then both hands together. He continued using the same procedure, increasing the speed to half-note tempo (two beats), followed by quarter-note (one beat), eighth-note (half beat), and sixteenth-note (quarter beat) tempos. Then he played chords and inversions in the same format. The process took two and a half hours. The stage manager asked Horowitz why he did not play some of his concert music. Vladimir explained that to play perfectly, one must practice perfectly. As my Physio-Synthesis teachers said, "You can never do the work too slow."

Our goal is to practice the movements correctly so that we will be able to (as described by Moshe Feldenkrais) "make the impossible possible, the possible easy, and the easy elegant." One major focus of the Dailey Inner Core Workout is to strengthen core and surface muscles and to secure joints in an anchoring mode, ready for action.

Normally, no more than three repetitions are performed in succession. If there are more than three, the newly recruited muscle fibers tend to fatigue, the stronger outer muscles take over, and the mind tends to wander. One day, a student brought her preschool-age daughter with some of her toys to class. When the class began, the little girl stopped playing with her toys and watched. She was curious and totally focused during the first three repetitions. Then I tested the importance of the three-repetition plan by adding one or two repetitions to several different movements. After the third repetition of every movement, she was not interested and went back to playing with her toys, but when a different movement began, she immediately stopped playing and watched the class. Evidently, the mind does begin to wander after three repetitions.

The first repetition is performed primarily by your surface muscles and does not use the inner core support. During the second rep, the outer muscles begin to let go of tension and your core muscles begin to come into action. During this rep, the weaker core and stronger surface muscles alternate and may produce jerky, wobbly movements.

Muscle cramps are another common occurrence that may happen during any repetition. As movements progress, weaker core muscles may become fatigued, causing them to cramp. Reverse the movement to give them a rest. This will allow the overly contracted muscles to relax, and the movement can be resumed with less force. As the muscles strengthen, the cramps will disappear. However, if these core muscles are inactive longer than two days, the muscles will begin to atrophy and cramps will return.

With stronger muscles, during the third repetition, the inner core muscles will initiate the movement rather than the surface muscles, resulting in a slower, smoother, and more uniform movement. With a regular workout plan, your core and surface muscles will be able to sustain a precise movement throughout and take it into everyday activities, and your inner core muscles will be able to initiate every movement.

A pause is vital to the successful completion of any repetition in order for the brain to retain a strong connection to the newly activated muscle fibers. During the pause, which may be the most unstable part of a repetition, some key points must be reinforced: increase stability, release excess tension, and maintain the objective. Compare the pause to the process after food intake and digestion before the body cells are able to absorb nutrients. With these things in mind, I'll walk you through the following exercises at beginning, intermediate, and advanced levels.

LEVEL KEY:

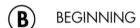 BEGINNING

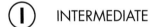 INTERMEDIATE

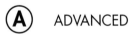 ADVANCED

Foot Movements—Triangle 1

Objectives: To strengthen ankles and the arches of your feet by balancing muscle pairs that flex and extend the foot, tilt the ankles inward and outward, and develop parallel foot alignment, placing the Achilles tendon behind the second and third toes and weight on the inner three metatarsals *(fig. 18)*. It is important for your feet to remain balanced and active in every weight-bearing movement. Narrow hips are usually impossible if weight is placed on the fifth metatarsal and your foot's outer border.

You will balance and reshape the muscle pair of inner and outer calf muscles. When your knees, toes, and toe joints are together, your inner calf muscles will also be together and there will be two spaces below the knees. One space will be above the ankles, and the other space between the calf muscles and knees. By strengthening your inner thigh, core abdominal, and hip muscles, you'll develop flat abdominals and narrow hips.

Anchoring Position—Sitting: Sit on a mat with your legs extended and at a right angle to your torso, hands on the mat below your shoulders, weight on your sit bones and the backs of your heels, your inner thigh and knee muscles active with your knees together. Active core knee joint muscles feel like a fist. Center the kneecaps upward. Lift your ribs upward from your hips to lengthen the spine. Your shoulders reach backward, downward, and outward.

Keep your arms long, palms down, fingers forward, collarbones wide, and your shoulder blades flat against your ribs. Center your head over your shoulders and ischium bones (sit bones). Reach the backs of your ears away from your shoulders.

Anchoring Position—Supine: Lie supine on a mat. Keep your great toes and toe joints together, heels approximately two and a half inches apart, Achilles tendon behind the midline of your forefoot (the space between your second and third toes). Tilt your feet inward to lift the outer arches. Feel your hips narrow and your core inner thighs and abdominals engage. Place your knees together, unlocked and centered. Tilt your pelvis back to place your SI joint dimples against the mat with balanced inner thighs, core abdominals, narrow hips, lengthened lumbar curve, and the L1-T23 apex anchored.

FIGURE 18

foot movements

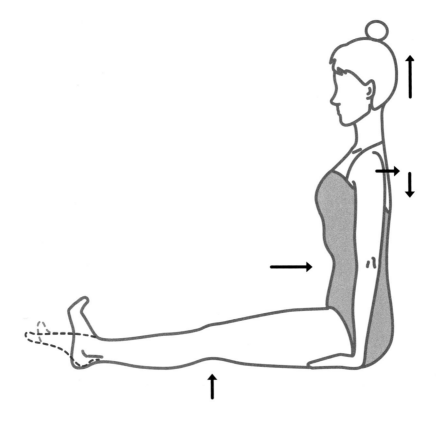

Feel narrowed hips, activated inner thighs, a toned gluteal fold, and a core abdominal hollow. Point your sit bones toward your heels and your knees forward, away from your head. Feel your core muscles from your knees to pelvis.

Reach the top of your sternum (breastbone) toward the ceiling and your head, with the low end of your sternum toward the mat and your feet, which will anchor the L1-T12 apex and level the sternum. Keep your collarbones wide, shoulder blades flat against the mat, back ribs down toward your waist and hollow below your front ribs. Feel your core shoulder girdle muscles. Reach your chin toward your sternum, the backs of your ears away from your shoulders, and the crown of your head away from your feet. Feel the cranial muscles of your head activate and give you a facelift.

Keep your arms long, palms down, fingers forward, and elbows unlocked and turned outward to open your elbow windows. This position of the elbows strengthens triceps, latissimus dorsi, and rotator cuff muscles. If your shoulder blades do not lie flat on the mat, then rounded shoulders, winging shoulder blades, and forward head position are the problem. In supine position, your collarbones will get assistance from gravity to release tension and widen your collarbones. For additional assistance, turn your palms upward. Feel your collarbones widen, allowing your shoulder blades to lay flat on the mat. Due to rounded shoulder and forward head posture habits, the cervical spine will be tight and short, causing the chin to lift up toward the ceiling. It may be necessary to place magazines, books, or other items under your head to raise it high enough to allow the chin to reach toward the sternum while keeping the opening of the ear horizontal.

The upper torso goal in supine position is to have your shoulder blades flat, arms long with palms down, elbows turned outward, and your head on the mat with the opening of your ears horizontal. The goal for standing is to have broad shoulders and to keep your neck long, your chin toward your sternum, and your head level.

Perform Foot Positions 1, 2, 3, 4, and 5, beginning with the right foot followed by the left foot, until the body-mind connection is familiar with the movement. When so, perform the movements with both feet in unison. Foot Positions 4 and 5 are similar to Positions 1 and 2, except that as the feet return to the beginning position, a corrective change takes place.

FOOT POSITION 1

Inhale toward your lower back and side ribs. Exhale to begin movement.

Lengthen the toes of your right foot downward, causing the knuckles to softly protrude. Keep toes long. Maintain feet tilting inward and keep ankles soft, unlocked, and at the ready. Repeat this movement with your left foot. Feel sole of foot muscle activity building strength and padding to prevent tender feet. Feel muscle connections between your feet, calves, thighs, abdominals, and up through your core to your cranial muscles. Feel your core abdominal hollow below your front ribs and your hip-narrowing muscles. Relax your toes.

Pause for muscle memory retention.

Reinforce Supine Anchoring Position to increase neuro-muscular reeducation. Relax your toes, and feel partial release of the muscle connection from your feet to your head. Inhale toward your lower back and side ribs to assist lengthening and widening of the lumbar vertebrae. Exhale to begin the movement.

FOOT POSITION 2

Turn the toes on your right foot up. Repeat the movement with your left foot. Feel the arches of your feet lift. Feel the muscle connection to your calves, thighs, and core abdominal hollow below your front ribs and the narrowing of your hips.

Tilt your feet inward to lift the outer arches, and place your little toes higher than the great toes. Feel the muscle connection extend from your feet to your head skullcap muscles, and feel your nasal passages open.

Pause for muscle memory retention.

Reinforce Supine Anchoring Position: Inhale toward your lower back and side ribs.

FOOT POSITION 3

Keep your toes turned up with your knees level and together. Maintain placement of your right forefoot on the right side of the midline as you reach the right ankle inward and lead with the little toes to flex the foot and lengthen the Achilles tendon. Repeat the movement with your left foot. Moving one foot at a time allows the brain to learn from the right foot and provides a better awareness of how to isolate the movement at the left ankle. Maintain unlocked, level knees to prevent borrowing length from the back of your knees rather than your Achilles. Feel your core abdominal hollow muscles below your front ribs.

Point the inside of your heels away from your sit bones, and pull your toes toward your head. Feel the muscle connection go through your feet to your cranial muscles. Feel the core-narrowing muscles of your hips.

Pause for muscle memory retention.

Reinforce Supine Anchoring Position: Notice the distance between your ankles. Inhale toward your lower back and side ribs.

FOOT POSITION 4

A very important corrective movement progression occurs when moving from Position 3 to 4. The neuromuscular re-education goal is to create less space between the ankles, the apex of Triangle I, while the heels remain apart. The right foot begins with your toes turned up. A strong foundation of core muscles will develop when your right ankle reaches inward as the inner, largest metatarsal slowly reaches away from your knees to softly lengthen your forefoot. Feel the movement lift your little toe metatarsal and the outer arch and strengthen arch support for your foot. Feel your core hip-narrowing muscles. Keep your toes turned up. Feel the muscle connection go through your feet to your cranium. Repeat the movement with your left foot. Activate core knee fist muscles to unlock your knees and ankles in order to maintain their strength and shock absorber duties. Notice: did the movement bring your ankles closer together than in Position 3?

Pause for muscle memory retention.

Reinforce Supine Anchoring Position. Inhale toward your lower back and side ribs. Feel the core abdominal hollow below your front ribs.

FOOT POSITION 5

Relax your toes. Feel a release in the muscle connections from your feet to your core abdominal muscles. Foot Position 5 looks like Position 1, except that your ankles are closer together, with your heels apart, due to the correction of the foot movement from Position 3 to Position 4.

Keep your toes lengthened as they reach downward with your metatarsal bones visible and your ankles reaching inward. Feel the muscles of your feet and their connection to your cranium. If you do not feel the connection, are your knees or ankles locked? If your spine is shorter with more curvature at the back of your neck or waist in supine position, you have lost length and core-anchoring muscles. If your knees or ankles are locked or if there is more curvature at the back of your neck or waist, the muscle connection will not go through to your head.

Repetitions: Three with your right and left feet working together in unison.

Hints for Beginners: The sitting position provides a visual as well as kinesthetic experience for beginners. Keep your ankles turned inward, little toes highest, outer arches lifted, knees together and level.

Supine Arm Option: Palms of your hands up with arms diagonal to your shoulders to widen your collarbones and flatten your shoulder blades.

Variation: Anchoring Position—Standing.

FOOT POSITION 3—STANDING

With your hands on the back of a chair, ballet bar, or wall for balance, place your heels apart *(fig. 19)*. Inhale toward your lower back and side ribs. Feel your core abdominal hollow below your front ribs. Exhale to begin movement. Sway forward from the heels with weight on your great, second, and third metatarsals to lift your heels into Foot Position 2. Reach your ankles inward to shift your weight inward; lift your outer foot arches and little toe metatarsals. Point your sit bones toward your heels to narrow your hips. Feel your inner thigh and hip-narrowing muscles.

Pause for muscle memory retention.

Reinforce Standing Anchoring Position. Inhale toward your lower back and side ribs. Feel your core abdominal hollow muscles.

Return to Foot Position 3. Press weight into your great metatarsals, reach your knees away from your head, and slowly lower your heels to the floor as your ankles reach inward, keeping your heels apart and weight on the inner half of your heels. The downward progression activates a deeper core layer of your inner thigh muscles. Feel increased inner

FIGURE 19
forward heel raises

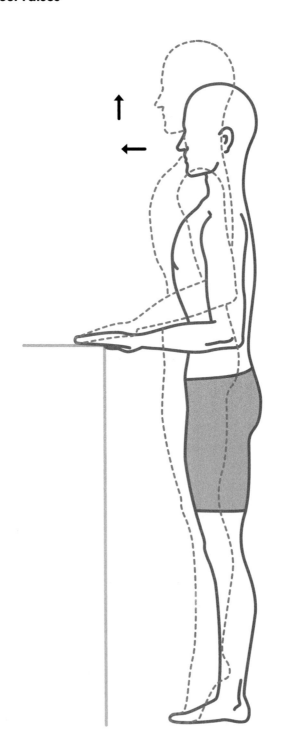

and outer calf, inner and outer thigh, hip-narrowing, and core abdominal muscles.

Repetitions: Three.

Variation: Sitting on a chair.

Movement: Same as Standing.

Leg Rotations—Triangle 2

Objectives: To develop a balance between the core and surface muscle layers that rotate your legs outward and the partners that rotate your legs inward. Balance your muscles in front with partners in the backs of your legs. Strengthen knee muscles to prevent locking and allow knee joints to function as stabilized shock absorbers. You will also strengthen your ankle and hip joints. Your inner core hip muscles are essential to narrowing your hips and allow centering of the knee joints. This activity also corrects shortened leg and hip joint dysfunction.

Anchoring Position: The positions are the same as foot movements. Sit on a mat for beginning or intermediate use. Lie supine on a mat for intermediate or advanced use (see pages 103 & 105). Remember the importance of anchoring apex L1-T12 in supine position.

FOOT POSITION 1

Lie supine on a mat. Inhale toward your lower back and side ribs *(fig. 20)*. Feel your core abdominal hollow below your front ribs. Exhale to begin the movement. Lengthen your toes downward, causing knuckles to be visible, and tilt your feet inward if possible. Feel the sole of your foot muscles, calves, thighs, core abdominals, and the muscle connection from your feet to your head. Slowly rotate your legs outward.

Pause for muscle memory retention.

Reinforce Supine Anchoring Position. Stabilize the pelvis in neutral, anchor L1-T12, and lengthen your spine. Inhale

FIGURE 20

leg rotations

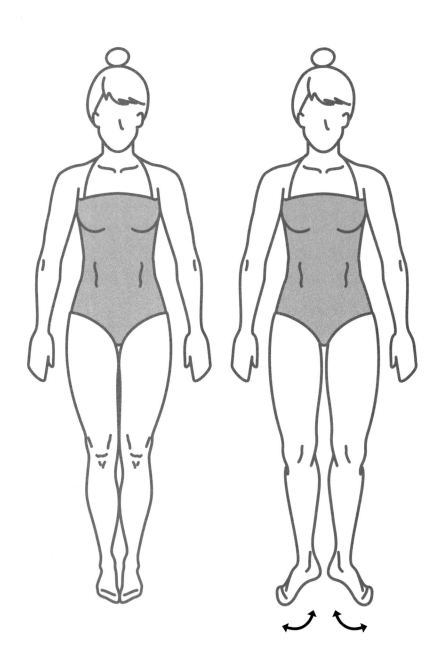

toward your lower back and side ribs. Feel your core abdominal hollow below the front ribs. Exhale to begin the movement.

Maintain the leg position with your toes long and reaching downward from the metatarsals. Move only the feet at the ankles as you reach the great metatarsals (ball of foot bones) inward and lift your lateral arches upward, creating a sling of support for the arches of the feet. Feel a pull under the great metatarsals, along with stronger inner thighs and the low abdominal muscle connection to the peroneus longus (muscles of your outer ankle).

Reach your knees toward your feet to unlock and activate your knee fist muscles. Feel the stabilization of your knee joints and a deeper activation of inner thigh and core abdominal muscles.

Think of your legs as logs. Maintain the alignment of your feet, ankles, and knees, as the ankles slowly lead the inward rotation of your legs to return the great toes, ankles, and knees together. To maintain the connection from your feet to your head, your ankles must arrive before your toes. Feel your hips narrow and your inner thigh and low abdominal muscles grow stronger.

Repetitions: Two.

FOOT POSITION 2

Reinforce Anchoring Position and Foot Position 1. Inhale toward your lower back and side ribs. Feel your core abdominal hollow below your front ribs. Relax your toes, and feel the muscles of your feet, foreleg, thighs, hips, and pelvis relax, along with a partial release of the muscle connection from your feet to your head. Exhale to begin the movement.

Turn your toes upward, and tilt your feet inward. Feel the muscles of your feet lift your arches. Feel the increase of calf, thigh, and abdominal muscles. Slowly rotate your legs outward.

Pause for muscle memory retention.

Reinforce Supine Anchoring Position and Foot Position 2. Inhale toward your lower back and side ribs. Anchor L1-T12. Feel your core abdominal hollow below your front ribs. Exhale to begin the movement.

Reach the great metatarsals away from your head and the little toe side of your feet toward your head to maintain the lift of your outer arches. Feel more core abdominals and the lifting action of your peroneus longus muscles from under the great metatarsals to the outer ankles and lateral side of your knees.

Tighten the fist muscles of your knee joint. Imagine pointing your knees away from your hips to get a stronger abdominal connection. Feel stabilization of your knee joints, deeper activation of your inner thigh, and core abdominal muscles.

Your ankles slowly lead the inward rotation of the legs to bring your great toes, toe joints, and knees together. Your ankles arrive before your toes. Feel your inner thigh, low abdominal, and hip-narrowing muscles gain strength. Feel the muscle connection from your feet to your head.

Repetitions: Two.

FOOT POSITION 3

Inhale toward your lower back and side ribs. Feel the hollow below your front ribs. Exhale to begin the movement. To progress from Foot Position 2 to 3, keep your toes turned up. Maintain placement of your right forefoot on the right side of the midline as you reach your ankle inward to flex the foot and lengthen behind the right heel. If the Achilles is tight, the right knee may lift slightly to "borrow length" for the right foot to be able to flex, but maintain your right knee level with your left knee. Repeat the movement with your left foot. Keep both knees level. Feel the front of your shin muscles strengthen and your Achilles lengthen. Feel the muscle connection go through to your head as your heels reach away from your hips and the toes pull toward your hips.

Maintain the reach with your heels, and pull your toes toward your hips as you slowly rotate your legs outward.

Pause for muscle memory retention.

Reinforce Anchoring Position and Foot Position 3.

Inhale toward your lower back and side ribs. Feel the hollow below your front ribs. Exhale to begin the movement. With your knees unlocked, reach your heels away from your head and pull your toes toward your head, lengthening behind your toes, ankles, knees, hips, waist, and neck. Also, reach your ankles inward and lift the lateral arches upward to maintain a lift of the lateral arches of your feet. Feel a pull under your great metatarsals, peroneus longus, and core abdominal muscles.

To activate fist muscles of your knee joints, reach your knees away from your hips. Feel stabilization of your knee joints and a deeper activation of your inner thigh and core abdominal muscles.

Maintain alignment of your feet, ankles, and knees. Remember to keep your legs like logs as your ankles slowly lead the inward leg rotation, and bring the great toes, toe joints, and inner knees together. Your ankles arrive before the toes. Feel your inner thigh, low abdominal, and hip-narrowing muscles grow stronger. Feel the muscle connection go from your feet (body foundation) through your body to your head.

Repetitions: Two.

FOOT POSITION 4

Inhale toward your lower back and side ribs. Feel the hollow below your front ribs. Exhale to begin the movement. Start with your right foot. Keep your toes lifted and on the right side of the midline. Reach your right ankle inward as the great metatarsal moves away from the knees to softly point the foot and lift the outer arch higher. Soften locked joints at your ankles and knees. Repeat the same movement with your left foot.

Maintain your ankles, reaching inward, outer arches and toes lifted as your legs slowly rotate outward.

Pause for muscle memory retention.

Reinforce Anchoring Position and Foot Position 4 with your toes turned up. Inhale toward your lower back and side ribs. Feel the hollow below your front ribs. Exhale to begin the movement.

Increase the action of your great metatarsals, reaching away from your hips and lifting up the outer arch toward your hips. Feel the pull under your great metatarsals, increased strength in the peroneus longus muscles, hip-narrowing, and your core abdominal hollow muscles.

Reach your knees away from your hips to activate the fist muscles of your knees. Feel stabilization of your knee joints, inner thighs, and core abdominal muscles. Maintain alignment of your feet, ankles, and knees as the ankles slowly lead the inward rotation of the legs, and bring together your great toes, ankles, and knees. Your heels remain apart. Feel your inner thigh, core low abdominal, and hip-narrowing muscles grow stronger.

Repetitions: Two.

FOOT POSITION 5

Inhale toward your lower back and side ribs. Feel the hollow below your front ribs. Exhale to begin the movement. Relax your toes. Feel the release in muscle connection from your feet to your core abdominals. Keep your ankles soft and toes long as your toes reach downward, causing your metatarsal bones to be visible. Feel the soles of your feet, calves, thighs, and abdominal muscles activate. Keep your ankles reaching inward as your legs slowly rotate outward.

Pause for muscle memory retention.

Reinforce Anchoring Position and Foot Position 5. Inhale toward your lower back and side ribs. Feel the hollow below your front ribs. Exhale to begin the movement. Increase the action of your great metatarsals, reaching away from your hip and lifting the outer arch toward your hip. Keep your toes long, with visible metatarsals. Feel the pull under your great metatarsals, increased strength in the peroneus longus muscle of your outer ankles, and your core abdominal muscle hollow below your front ribs. To activate your knee fists and abdominal muscles, reach your knees away from your hips. Feel stabilization of your knee joints and deeper activation of your inner thigh and core abdominal muscles.

Maintain alignment of your feet, ankles, and knees as your ankles slowly lead the inward rotation of your legs to bring together your great toes, ankles, and knees. Your heels remain apart. Keep reaching your knees toward your feet. Feel your inner thigh, core abdominal, and hip-narrowing muscles grow stronger.

Repetitions: Two.

Option: One Leg Rotation repetition from Foot Positions 1 through 5.

Hints for Beginners: The sitting position with legs extended provides a visual as well as kinesthetic experience for beginners, as you are able to see the movement you are asking your body to execute.

Hip Lift

Objectives: To develop strength and balance between your anterior and posterior surfaces and core spinal and shoulder girdle muscles. With your legs and hip joints at a right angle to your torso, your lumbar spine is naturally lengthened and stable.

Anchoring Position: Sit on a mat with your legs extended, great toes together in Foot Position 1, knees together and unlocked, hip joints at a right angle to your torso, and hands beside your hips, palms down with fingers softly placed together, pointing forward, and thumbs straight and under the lateral side of your gluteal muscles *(fig. 21)*.

Movement: After a Leg Rotation returns to the medial centerline, a Hip Lift may follow from Foot Positions 1 through 5. With elbows facing outward, maintain the position of keeping your shoulders back and down toward your "back jean pockets." Reach the backs of your ears away from your shoulders to lengthen your neck. Inhale toward your lower back and side ribs. Exhale, push the hands down into the mat to reach the spine upward, and lift your body weight from the sit bones. Depending upon the length of your arm to torso ratio, the sit bones and gluteal area will barely feel the mat or rise above it. If your torso is longer than your arms, magazines or blocks may be placed under your hands to add length to your arms. Feel your shoulder girdle muscle support.

Pause for muscle memory retention.

Maintain Foot Position 1 and slowly lower your hips with your shoulders backward, downward, and reaching outward as the backs of your ears reach upward away from your shoulders. Prepare for Leg Rotations from Foot Position 2 and 3.

Repetitions: One, following a Leg Rotation.

Knee Spreads—Triangle 2

Three different knee spreads develop the six layers of inner thigh muscles. Narrow Spreads activate surface layers (five

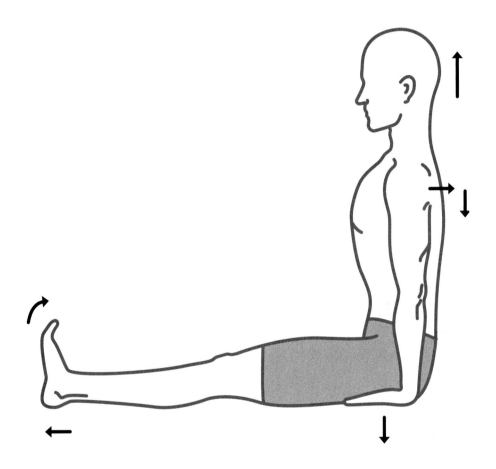

FIGURE 21

hip lift

and six). Medium Spreads activate middle layers (three and four). Sprawls (wide spreads) activate deep core layers (one and two) of the inner thighs as well as core hip outer rotator muscles.

Objectives: To balance six muscles at your hip joints that rotate your thighs inward with six muscle partners that rotate your thighs outward; balance surface, middle, and core layers of inner thigh muscles; build support for your sacrum and spinal column; narrow hips; strengthen your pelvic floor muscles; balance the alignment of your pelvis to assist in the prevention of knee, hip, back, rib, and neck problems.

Anchoring Position: Lie supine on a mat with your knees bent and feet standing parallel at a right angle to your foreleg, toes lifted, heels separated with your Achilles tendon behind the space between toes two and three, great toes and toe joints together, and lateral borders of your feet lifted to move your ankles toward the midline *(fig. 22)*. Balance your weight over your arches between the great, second, and third toes and inner half of your heel with your knees together. Feel your hips narrow, your core inner thigh, and your low abdominal muscles.

Place the pelvis in neutral with your waistline rolled back to lengthen the front of your hips, and place your SI joint dimples flat on the mat to balance your lumbar curve. Point your sit bones toward your feet. Anchor L1-T12, the apex of Triangles 3 and 4, with the top of your breastbone toward the ceiling and your head, the bottom of your breastbone toward the mat and your feet. With both ends of the lumbar curve anchored (SI joint dimples and L1-T12), your body is secure for movement. There is a strong connection between the hips (Triangle 2) and shoulders (Triangle 4). The diagonal muscle connection of the right shoulder to left hip and the left shoulder to right hip must be in balance. The anchoring of L1-T12 thoracic vertebrae and broad shoulders are necessary to rebuild balanced alignment.

The shoulder position requires you to keep your collarbones wide, shoulder blades back and down toward your hips, and sternum (breastbone) in horizontal alignment as described above. Feel your core shoulder muscles and the hollow below your front ribs. With your chin toward your sternum and the backs of your ears and the crown of your head reaching away from your shoulders, you should feel facial muscles tone.

NARROW KNEE SPREADS

Inhale toward your lower back and side ribs. Feel the hollow below your front ribs. Exhale to begin the movement. Tilt your pelvis back toward the mat to lengthen the front of your hips and back of your waist. Feel your core muscles and the deeper hollow below your front ribs. With your chin toward your sternum and the backs of your ears reaching away from your shoulders, reach your knees away from your head. Feel muscle connections go through to open your nasal passages and tone your cranial muscles.

With the feet anchored and movement restricted between your ankles and hips, slowly spread your knees approximately two inches. You will feel a place where the inner thighs activate (surface muscle layers five and six). When Triangle 1 is secure with your ankles reaching inward, you will experience a feeling of resistance to opening the knees wider. Maintain the lift of your lateral arches with your little toes above the mat to maintain weight on the great, second, and third metatarsals and your ankles reaching inward. Feel your back ribs open as your knees spread.

Pause for muscle memory retention.

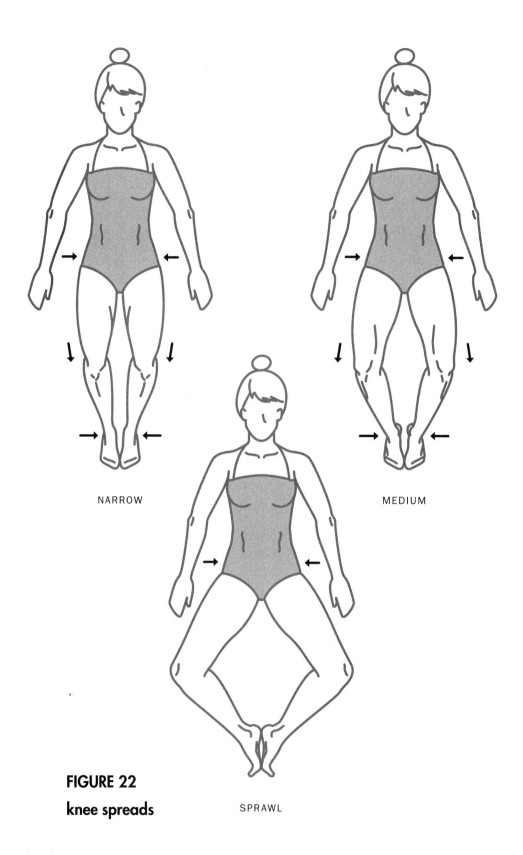

NARROW

MEDIUM

SPRAWL

FIGURE 22
knee spreads

Reinforce Supine Anchoring Position and Feet Standing Position. Inhale toward your lower back and side ribs. Feel the hollow below your front ribs. Exhale to begin movement.

Reach your knees away from your head, and slowly bring your knees together. Feel increased activity of your inner knee, thigh, hip-narrowing, core abdominal, and cranial muscles. These muscles will not be active unless your pelvis is tilted backward with your waist and L1-T12 on the mat.

Repetitions: Three.

Hints for Beginners: Keep your arms in a diagonal line from your shoulders with your palms upward.

MEDIUM KNEE SPREADS

Anchoring and movement are the same as Narrow Knee Spreads, except the spread is wider (approximately hip-width apart, middle muscle layers three and four). Tilt your pelvis back toward the mat to lengthen the front of your hips and back of your waist. With your toes lifted, ankles anchored reaching inward, and movement restricted between your ankles and hips, slowly spread your knees. Feel the Narrow Spread limit and pause. Slowly spread the knees wider until you experience another feeling of resistance. Feel this Medium Spread limit. Pause, reach your knees away from your head, and slowly bring your knees together. Feel your core inner thigh, abdominal hollow, and core hip-narrowing muscles. These muscles will not be active unless your pelvis is tilted backward with your waist and L1-T12 anchored on the mat.

Repetitions: Three.

SPRAWLS

Anchoring is the same as for Narrow and Medium Knee Spreads. Feel the activation of your facial muscles and the muscle connection through to the opening of your nasal passages. Tilt your pelvis back toward the mat to lengthen the front of your hips and back of your waist. With your toes lifted, ankles anchored reaching inward, and movement restricted between your ankles and hips, slowly spread your knees. Feel Narrow Spread limit and pause. Slowly spread the knees wider, feel Medium Spread limit, and pause. Keep your toes lifted, and slowly open your legs and feet outward into a diamond shape as the soles of your feet come together.

Relax pelvis and toes. Press the soles of your feet together. Feel your pelvic floor muscles. Release the press. Lift your toes, and press the sides of your feet into the mat. Feel the deepest hip-narrowing muscles (layers one and two).

Pause for muscle memory retention.

Reinforce pelvic tilt, and keep your toes lifted. Inhale toward your lower back and side ribs. Feel your back ribs broaden. Feel your abdominal hollow. Exhale to begin movement. Reach your knees away from your head. With toes lifted, slowly reach your great toes, toe joints, ankles, and knees inward to bring your feet to standing and anchoring position. Again, reach the knees away from your head. Feel your face lift and the muscle connection through your abdominals to your nasal passages.

Repetitions: Three.

Leg Spreads—Triangle 2

Objectives: To strengthen midline support of your core muscle and joint action through your body from your feet to the crown of your head. All triangles must be secure to feel the connection of muscle participation through your whole body.

Anchoring Position: Lie prone on a mat with great toes and knees together *(fig. 23)*. Press your pubic bone down, and point your sit bones toward your heels to lengthen the front

FIGURE 23

leg spreads

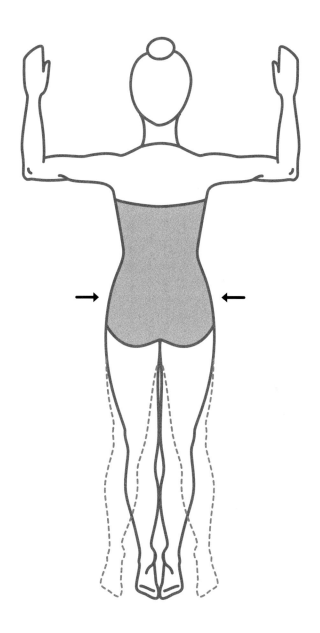

of your hips and lumbar spine. Feel activation of your gluteal and hip-narrowing muscles. Relax your toes. Point and tilt your feet inward, placing the outer borders and little toes on the mat—the opposite of supine position. Keep your heels apart as your ankles reach inward. Press your forehead gently into the mat.

Movement: Reach your knees toward your feet to activate knee fist, core inner thigh, and abdominal muscles. Keep a straight line from your great toes, inner ankles, and knees as the legs spread apart against an imaginary resistance.

Pause for muscle memory retention.

Release surface abdominal and gluteal tension. Reinforce anchoring position and prevent knees from turning outward. Use core muscles to bring your toes, toe joints, ankles, knees, and inner thighs together against an imaginary resistance. Remember, your ankles must arrive before your toes. Feel the muscle connection from your feet to your head.

Repetitions: Three.

Variation: Supine with legs extended.

Pelvic Tilts & Lifts—Triangle 3

Objectives: To create a balance between all of the muscle pairs that line the spine. These movements strengthen weak muscles of the vertebrae lining your spine on the anterior side of your waist and neck and lengthen tense muscles lining your spine on the posterior side of your waist and neck, lengthening the spine from one end to the other. Pelvic movements strengthen core abdominals, narrow hips, and tone your gluteal muscles.

Anchoring Position: Lie supine on a mat with knees bent and feet standing in Triangle 1 position *(fig. 24)*. With your knees together, tilt your feet inward to lift your outer arches. Lift your toes to activate muscles of your calves, thighs, and hips.

FIGURE 24
pelvic tilts and lifts

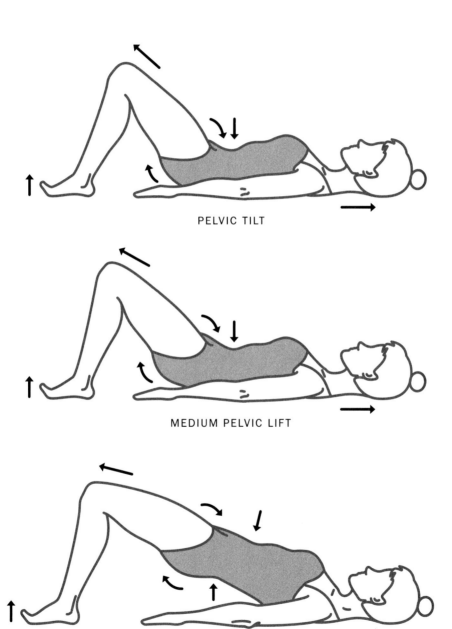

PELVIC TILT

MEDIUM PELVIC LIFT

BRIDGE

Position your pelvis in neutral with both ends of the lumbar curve anchored; keep SI joint dimples and the L1-T12 apex on the mat. Reach your chin toward your sternum and the backs of your ears away from your shoulders to anchor your head and maintain the length of your neck.

(B) PELVIC TILT

Think of your spine as a hammock anchored at your head and hips. When the pelvis tilts backward, placing the back of your waist on the mat, the pubic bone turns upward. This lengthens your lumbar spine, inner thighs, and anterior hip psoas (hip stabilizers). Your core abdominal and gluteal muscles are strengthened. As your tailbone and lower sacrum lift above the mat, your low spine is lengthened into the shape of a hammock.

Pause for muscle memory retention.

Reinforce Supine Anchoring Position: To test for surface pelvic tension, squeeze your gluteal muscles and feel the surface gluteal muscles contract. Release the squeeze. Feel your surface muscles let go and your core muscles activate. Inhale toward your lower back and side ribs to anchor the L1-T12 apex. Maintain open ribs as you exhale. Slowly lower your SI joint dimples and sacrum to the mat, placing your pelvis in neutral. Feel your core inner thigh, abdominal hollow, anchored L1-T12 apex, and hip-narrowing muscles.

Repetitions: Beginning, use three. Reduce to two and one repetitions in intermediate and advanced use. All Pelvic Lifts have the same basic objectives and Anchoring Position.

(B) MEDIUM PELVIC LIFT

Turn your toes up, heels apart, and ankles inward. Press your knees together, and reach your knees away from your hips to tip your pubic bone up and lengthen the front of your hips. Roll your waist back to the mat into a pelvic tilt to lengthen your lumbar spine. Maintain your head anchored with your chin toward your breastbone and the backs of your ears reaching away from your shoulders. As you add more tilt to the pelvis, reach your knees away from your head to feel core knee fist and abdominal muscles. Slowly lift the spine one vertebra at a time. Anchor your head, add more tilt to your pelvis, and reach your knees away from your head as each vertebra of the spine lifts until it reaches the vertebra at the lower edge of your shoulder blades. Keep your shoulder blades flat on the mat.

Pause for muscle memory retention.

Inhale toward your lower back and side ribs to anchor your L1-T12 apex. Exhale, let your sternum sink heavily toward the mat, and slowly lower your spine one vertebra at a time. Anchor your head, add more tilt to the pelvis, and reach your knees away from your head to maintain length of the spine as each vertebra rolls down and returns to a pelvic tilt. Inhale toward your lower back and side ribs to anchor your L1-T12 apex. Exhale, and slowly lower your SI joint dimples and sacrum to the mat, placing your pelvis in neutral. Feel your core inner thigh, abdominal hollow, anchored L5-T12 apex, and hip-narrowing muscles.

BRIDGE

Place your toes together, heels apart and ankles inward, and press your knees together. Reach your knees away from your head to tip up the pubic bone, lengthen the back of your waist and front of your hips, and activate your knee fist and abdominal muscles. Continue to reach your knees away from your head to level your hips and decompress the space inside the hip sockets. Stabilize your head with your chin toward your breastbone, with the backs of your ears reaching away from your shoulders as you add more tilt to the pelvis. Add a tilt, and reach as the spine lifts one vertebra at a time into a diagonal line from your knees to your hips and shoulders while maintaining the lumbar spine in neutral.

Pause for muscle memory retention.

Inhale toward your lower back and side ribs. Exhale, and slowly lower your spine one vertebra at a time. As your spine returns, anchor your L1-T12 apex and SI joint dimples when they reach the mat to place your pelvis into balanced neutral alignment and achieve a natural lumbar arch at the back of your waist. Feel your core inner thigh, abdominal hollow, anchored L1-T12, cranial, gluteal, and hip-narrowing muscles.

 LOW PELVIC LIFT

Gently press the inner three metatarsals of your feet into the mat. Inhale, maintaining awareness of your broad back ribs at the L1-T12 apex. Exhale, and reach your knees away from your head and the backs of your ears away from your feet to slightly lift your spine without arching or sagging at the waistline. Feel your spine lengthen.

Pause for muscle memory retention.

Release tension. Maintain the level of your hips and ears; reach your knees to lengthen your spine, narrow your hips, and create backward placement of the ribs at L1-T12. Slowly lower your spine all in one piece. The release of tension is a sign of inner control. Feel your core inner thigh and abdominal hollow muscles. Secure L1-T12 and your cranial, gluteal, and hip-narrowing muscles.

Head Lifts—Triangle 5

Objectives: To lift your head without arching the cervical spine, center your head position above your shoulders and lengthen your posterior neck muscles in order to tone your anterior neck muscles. You will perform three levels of head lifts, beginning with High, followed by Medium and Low. The High Head Lift is for beginning use due to the lighter weight of the head when it is lifted closer to the vertical (light line) of gravity. These movements gradually create a balance of strength with flexibility of the four layers of anterior and posterior core and surface muscles of your neck *(fig. 25)*.

HIGH HEAD LIFT

(B)

Lie supine on a mat with your knees bent, feet standing, heels apart, ankles inward, toes up, shoulders back and down toward your "back jean pockets," chin toward your sternum, and the backs of your ears away from your shoulders. Reach your knees away from your head to roll your waist back into a pelvic tilt. Inhale toward your lower back and side ribs to anchor your L1-T12 apex. Exhale to begin movement. Lead with your forehead as you lift your head and look toward your knees.

Pause for muscle memory retention.

Release tension of your surface abdominal six-pack. Maintain your shoulders back and down away from your ears, your lower back ribs wide with your L1-T12 apex anchored. Notice your shoulders. If they lift upward, your chin also has a tendency to lift and your benefits are lost. Reinforce your pelvic tilt. Reach your knees away from your hips, and feel your inner core muscle connection go through your knees to your head. Lead with the back of your neck to lower your head. With your head and L1-T12 apex anchored, lower your SI joint dimples to the mat, placing your lumbar spine in neutral. Lower your toes.

A Pelvic Lift may precede or follow the Head Lift. As your Head Lift movements progress to a lower height and the force of gravity increases, your inner core muscles gradually increase in strength and your cervical spine lengthens.

MEDIUM HEAD LIFT

Relax your surface neck muscles. With your heels apart, ankles reaching inward, and your toes lifted, reach your knees

FIGURE 25
head lifts

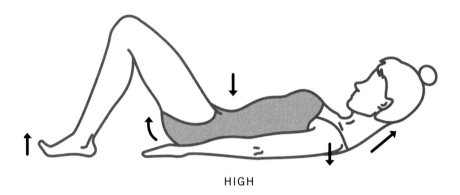

HIGH

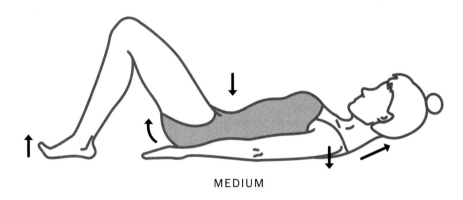

MEDIUM

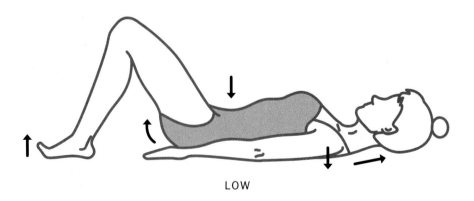

LOW

away from your head to roll your waist back into a pelvic tilt. Inhale toward your lower back and side ribs to anchor your L1-T12 apex. Release your surface abdominal six-pack muscles, and feel the action of your inner core muscles as you exhale and lift your head upward into medium height while maintaining length at back of your neck.

Pause for muscle memory retention.

Maintain your shoulders back and down toward your back jean pockets, the L1-T12 apex secure, and reach your knees away from your head as your lengthened cervical curve leads to lower your head. With your head and the L1-T12 apex anchored, lower your SI joint dimples to the mat and lower your toes. Feel your muscles relax.

LOW HEAD LIFT

With your toes lifted, ankles reaching inward, shoulders anchored back and down toward your back jean pockets, your chin toward your sternum, and the backs of your ears away from your shoulders, reach your knees away from your head to roll your waist back into a pelvic tile. Slightly lift your head above the mat while maintaining your balanced, lengthened cervical curve.

Pause for muscle memory retention.

Secure all joints. Lower your head with the support of your core cervical and lumbar spinal muscles.

Reversals of the Spine & Neck—Triangles 3, 4, 5, & 6

Physical discomfort is often the result of repeated misuse over a long period of time, caused by unevenly distributed weight within our body structure when standing, sitting, or walking inefficiently. The common cause results from tense surface muscles in the back of the neck, front of shoulders, and back of the waist, partnered with overstretched muscles behind the shoulders and in front of the neck and waist.

Tense and overstretched muscles block the inner support of core muscles on the anterior and posterior sides of the spine. The absence of outer tension is a sign of inner core control.

Reversals redevelop five areas of the spine. The first reversal is at the top (the neck), the second is at the waistline, the third is between the shoulders, the fourth is at the pelvic floor, and the fifth reverses the entire spine.

Reversal movements cannot be performed accurately until core muscle strength has developed to sufficiently anchor both ends of the spine and provide a stable foundation. In order to provide the stabilization required, precede and follow all reversals with a Pelvic Lift followed by a Head Lift.

Objectives: To balance the inner core and surface posterior and anterior vertebral muscles of your spine. Return to the natural balanced appearance of your first years, a smooth back without vertebrae of the spine protruding or sinking between tense surface muscles that parallel an indented spine. Reversals are also beneficial for the health and function of the body's nerves, organs, and glands, as well as improving abnormal curvatures of the spine.

Anchoring Position for Reversals: Lie supine on a mat with your knees bent and feet standing in Triangle 1 position. With your knees together, tilt your feet inward to lift your outer arches. Lift your toes to activate the muscles of your calves, thighs, and hips. Place your pelvis in neutral with both ends of your lumbar curve, SI joint dimples, and the L1-T12 apex anchored to the mat. Reach your chin toward your sternum and the backs of your ears away from your shoulders to anchor your head, and maintain the length of your neck. Feel the muscle connection from your toes through to your head.

Chin Lifts—Triangle 5

HIGH CHIN LIFT

(B)

Reach your knees away from your head to lengthen the front of your hips, and roll your waist back into a pelvic tilt (fig. 26) Anchor the L1-T12 apex. Slowly lift your chin, rotating your head upward at the atlas (first vertebra of the neck), which is level with your ears. As your chin lifts higher, be aware of the stopping point before your neck begins to increase its curve. Notice how the top of your sternum lifts, your collarbones widen, and your shoulder blades flatten against the mat. Reach the lower part of your sternum back to the mat and down toward your feet to reinforce anchoring of the L1-T12 apex and to maintain your inner core abdominal hollow below your front ribs.

Pause for muscle memory retention.

Reach your shoulders back, down toward your back jean pockets, and outward to broaden your shoulders and lengthen your neck while your chin stays lifted. Slowly lower your chin toward your sternum; reach the backs of your ears away from your shoulders and your knees away from your hips. With both ends of the spine lengthened in opposite directions, feel the muscle connection from your inner core hip-narrowing, abdominal-hollow, and shoulder-broadening muscles, along with the activated cranial muscles of your head that will lift your face and broaden your eyebrows and nasal passages. Chin Lifts help to tone saggy anterior neck muscles and lengthen the cervical curve. Maintaining length at the back of the neck allows oxygen to reach the back area of the throat, preventing bad breath and tonsil stones. Remember, if there is overlapping tissue forming a horizontal wrinkle on the back of the neck, a lack of oxygen there may cause a green skin microbiome to grow.

FIGURE 26
chin lifts

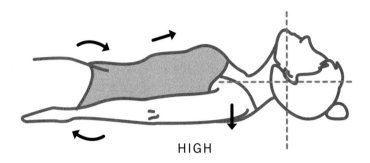

HIGH

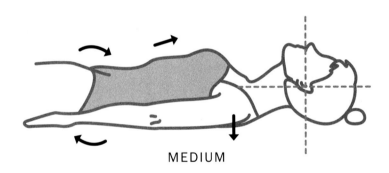

MEDIUM

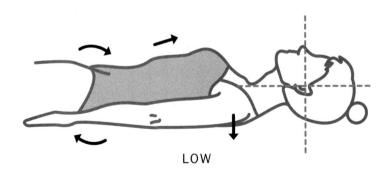

LOW

136

I first saw green growth on the back of a student's neck when she lengthened her cervical spine and opened the skin that was folded in her neck wrinkle.

MEDIUM CHIN LIFT

Anchor both ends of your spine. Reach your knees away from your hips to roll your waist back into a pelvic tilt as the backs of your ears reach away from your feet. Slowly lead with your eyebrows and forehead to raise your chin to a medium level. Feel the top of your sternum lift upward and toward your head as your shoulders broaden.

Pause for muscle memory retention.

Reinforce lengthened spine, narrowed hips, L1-T12 apex, and broadened shoulders anchoring positions. Release any surface muscle tension in your neck to allow the deepest inner core neck muscles that attach the spine to the skull to slowly replace your chin. Feel the core muscles of your neck and head lengthen your neck, broaden your shoulders, and tone your facial muscles. With stronger inner core muscle control, the movement will grow slower and smoother with less effort, and the position of your head and the contour of your neck will improve.

LOW CHIN LIFT

Anchor your pelvis in neutral with your hips narrow and shoulders broad. Reach your knees away from your head to anchor the L1-T12 apex, and roll your pelvis back into a tilt. Slightly raise your chin using only the deepest core anterior and posterior vertebral muscles that connect the head to the neck.

Pause for muscle memory retention.

Reinforce your heels apart and ankles inward with weight on your inner three metatarsals (ball of foot bones). Maintain weight on your spine from your low ribs and the

137

FIGURE 27

reversals

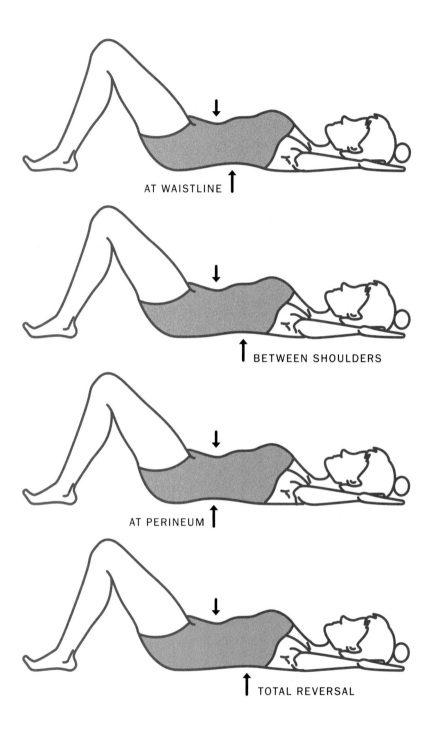

AT WAISTLINE

BETWEEN SHOULDERS

AT PERINEUM

TOTAL REVERSAL

L1-T12 apex to your waist and upper sacrum. Slowly reach the backs of your ears away from your shoulders to lengthen the back of your neck. Relax the surface muscles of your neck to allow your inner core neck muscles to slowly and effortlessly replace your chin.

Movement Options: Chin Lifts are advanced use when executed in Prone, Standing, and Cat-Spine Extended Positions. You must be able to maintain the pelvis in neutral and lift your chin without arching your lumbar spine.

Reversals—Triangles 3 & 4

REVERSAL AT WAISTLINE

Ⓑ

Unlike the lordosis (hyperextended, rooster tail) posture, which shortens the back of the waist *(fig. 6)* with surface muscles, this movement will be controlled by inner core spinal muscles. With your knees bent and feet standing on a mat, toes up and ankles inward, anchor both ends of your lumbar spine, the SI joint dimples at the lower end and L1-T12 apex at the upper end *(fig. 27)*. Place your arms in a diagonal position from your shoulders with your palms turned upward or downward near your hips. With your chin toward your sternum and the backs of your ears reaching away from your shoulders, gently press your head into the mat to maintain length at your neck. Reach your knees away from your head to lengthen the front of your hips and roll your waist back into a pelvic tilt. Slowly lift your lumbar spine upward with your waistline lightly touching the mat.

Pause for muscle memory retention.

Release tension of the surface spinal muscles near your waist to activate the deepest core posterior vertebral muscles. If you feel one side of the spine closer to the mat than the other, inhale and direct the breath toward the side that is higher. This will help release muscle tension and balance muscles on the opposite side of the spine.

Maintain your ankles inward, toes up, knees together, and your shoulders back and down toward your back jean pockets. With your inner core muscles, slowly and smoothly reach your knees away from your head to tip your pubic bone upward and replace your spine at the waistline with your SI joint dimples flat and your L1-T12 apex anchored.

Ⓘ REVERSAL BETWEEN SHOULDERS

With your knees bent and feet standing on the mat, your ankles inward and toes up, anchor your spine at both ends. Keep your hips narrow and your neck long and relaxed. Place your arms in a diagonal position near your hips with palms upward and thumbs and fingers touching the mat. Feel your shoulders open wide. Lift your sternum and chest upward to arch the thoracic spine between the shoulder blades with minimal shortening of the lumbar spine. The goal of this movement is to open your shoulders outward and back, flatten your shoulder blades, and release shoulder tension and spinal curvatures.

Pause for muscle memory retention.

Notice if the thoracic spine does not evenly arch upward. Inhale toward the tense half of the muscle pairs to balance both sides of the posterior back muscles with both sides of the chest. Keep the top of your sternum upward and toward your head and your shoulders back and outward. Slowly place the low end of the sternum backward and toward the feet as the pelvis rolls back into neutral position with your L1-T12 apex anchored, your SI joint dimples flat, and your spine lengthened.

Ⓘ REVERSAL AT PERINEUM

Reversal at the Perineum (pelvic floor) is initiated in the opposite direction of the pelvic tilt. It strengthens the inner core muscles to hold your pelvic girdle organs in their naturally

designated positions, as well as to prevent urinary incontinence and prolapsed organs.

With your knees bent and feet standing on a mat, your
ankles inward and toes up, anchor your spine at both ends
with the backs of your ears reaching away from your hips,
your shoulders back, down, and reaching outward, the L1-
T12 apex back to the mat, the SI joint dimples flat, and sit
bones reaching toward your feet. Slowly reach your knees
away from your head to roll your pelvis back into a pelvic
tilt. Secure the L1-T12 apex, and, with a very small and slow
movement, lower your pubic bone into the reversal position.

Pause for muscle memory retention.

Release surface muscle tension and feel the activation
of your core muscles, pelvic floor, and sacrum. With newly
found posterior and anterior inner core spinal muscle partners, slowly tilt your pubic bone upward to place your SI
joint dimples flat and your L1-T12 apex anchored in a balanced, neutral pelvis position.

TOTAL REVERSAL

All sections of the spine will be lifting together in Total Reversal (*fig. 27*). The movement is very slight and primarily
sensual rather than visible.

Reach the backs of your ears away from your shoulders
and reach sit bones toward your feet to lengthen both ends of
your spine. Reach your knees away from your hips to length-
en the front of your hips, and roll your waist back into a pelvic tilt. Feel your lower back ribs at the L1-T12 apex. With
core muscles of your spine ready for action, in a very slow
and small movement, lift all joints of your spine together in
unison with the vertebrae lightly touching the mat.

Pause for muscle memory retention.

Test the height of the reversal at your waist with a rul-
er. If it can slide under your spine, posterior surface spinal

muscles are overpowering anterior inner core muscle activation, causing an imbalance of the anterior surface and core muscles with the posterior surface and core muscles. Notice the balance of core right and left posterior muscles with core right and left anterior muscles. Inhale, and release tension. Exhale, and, with all joints together in action from your sacrum to your head, return the spine into a pelvic tilt.

(A) Cat Positions

Objectives: To create a balance of surface and core muscles between the anterior and posterior sides and between both ends of your spine. Structural support from your hands, arms, and shoulders, along with your knees, feet, legs, and hips, will activate all joints of your body, decompress spinal discs, and correct or minimize irregular lumbar curvatures.

Anchoring Position: Kneel on a mat with your knees and toe joints together, foreleg on mat, ankles inward with little toes, and outer borders of feet on a mat *(fig. 28)*. Tilt your pubic bone upward, hip points back, and sit bones away from your shoulders toward the back of your knees to lengthen the front of your hips and lumbar curve, narrow hips, tone gluteal muscles, and anchor your pelvis. Feel your inner core hollow and abdominal muscles when your sit bones reach toward your knees.

Place your hands on your thighs with your fingers softly together, thumbs at a right angle together at the midline in a goalpost shape with your elbows pointing outward. Slowly lift your arms to shoulder level. Bend forward from your hips. With your thumbs together, place your palms on the mat the same distance from your knees as your shoulders from your hips. To level your spine in a horizontal plane, reinforce your sit bones, reaching away from your head, the backs of your ears away from your shoulders and the low end of your sternum reaching toward the ceiling and away

FIGURE 28

cat positions

Keep shoulders broad and away from your ears.

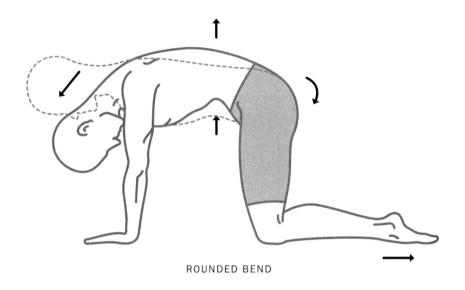

ROUNDED BEND

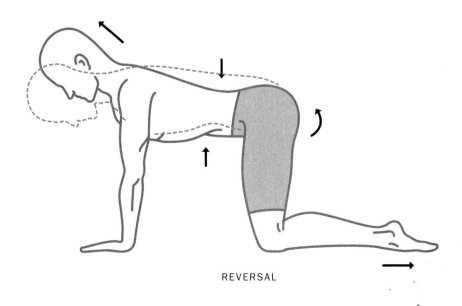

REVERSAL

from your shoulders as your upper sternum reaches toward the mat and your head.

With your ankles reaching inward, reach your shoulders outward to stabilize your shoulder joints. Slowly lift the back of your waist upward into a round bend. Maintain this position, and, in small movements, slowly sway backward and forward to release muscle tension and activate additional inner core muscles.

Pause for muscle memory retention.

Reinforce the round bend of the spine and back of neck, reaching away from your knees. Reach your ankles inward, and turn your elbows outward with your shoulders wide and away from your ears. Feel your stomach flatten and the strong muscle connection engage from your pelvis to your head.

With very small movements—to prevent surface muscles from blocking out your inner core muscles—slowly return into the flat back, tabletop position from your sit bones to the crown of your head. Begin at the pelvis and slowly lift your tail bone slightly upward, the upper end of your sternum upward, and reach the back of your neck away from the mat. Maintain collarbones wide with your elbows turned outward. Slowly sway backward and forward to feel the details of each joint.

Pause for muscle memory retention.

Now, with your back in neutral, tabletop position, explore your body's balanced muscle connection. Let your head and neck hang down, and feel the release of abdominal muscle contraction. Lead with the back of your neck to return your head to the flat-back position. Feel the abdominal muscles working and their connection to your head and neck. A postural, forward-headed position leads to saggy abdominals. Think of where your head is during the day, especially when you are at your computer.

Repetitions: Three. The second repetition reversal begins at the head-neck and travels downward to your tailbone. In the third repetition, the reversal involves every joint of the spine at the same time.

Shoulder Movements—Triangle 4

Objectives: Shoulders carry more tension than almost any other area of the body. During everyday activities such as sitting, talking on a cell phone, or working on a computer, the shoulders tend to round forward. Eventually, the neuromuscular system accepts tight, rounded shoulders as normal. Shoulder movements will help you unlearn this bad postural habit, rid harmful tension, and return your body into a well-aligned, balanced state. Many inner core and surface muscle pairs are involved.

Your shoulder and arm muscles are connected to your thorax (chest and ribs). Shoulder movements minimize rib imbalance from scoliosis, compressed ribs, and breathing problems. Improvement in your rib and shoulder-girdle alignment also improves alignment of your thoracic spine and sternum. When your shoulders broaden, your respiratory capacity improves as your shoulder blades flatten, hollows above your collarbones disappear, and your core rotator cuff and triceps muscles are strengthened.

Anchoring Position: Sit on a mat with your knees bent and feet standing in Triangle 1 position with your toes up and ankles reaching inward. Interlace your fingers, and wrap your hands below your knees with your elbows pointing outward *(fig. 29).* Slowly roll your waistline slightly backward, placing your neck, shoulders, and waist in a smooth, long outward curve. Awareness and stabilization of the L1-T12, apex of Triangles 3 and 4, is very important.

FIGURE 29

shoulder movements

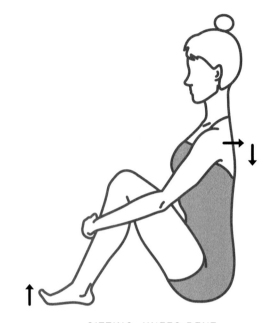

SITTING, KNEES BENT

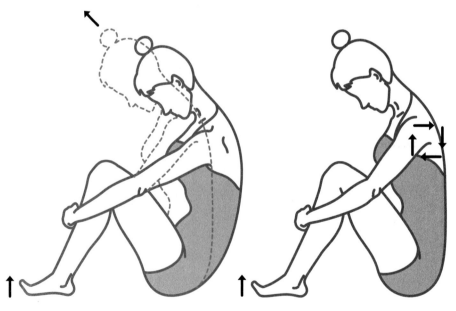

PREPARATION   UPWARD/DOWNWARD

146

POSITION 1

Inhale toward your lower back and side ribs. Exhale, and slowly lead your forehead and the top of your sternum to lean forward and up, with your eyes looking at your knees. Maintain the length of your neck, and, with a slow, small movement, lift your shoulders toward your ears. If you regularly carry tension in your shoulders, your brain may think this is a normal shoulder position. Continue, and slowly lift your shoulders as high as they will go toward your ears into a protective, "save the neck from danger" mode. By exaggerating tension in the muscles that lift your shoulder, your brain gets the signal that it is a temporary, protective action, and it accepts the promotion of reversing shoulder muscle tension. Feel the release of your low abdominal muscles as your shoulders' protective armor takes over.

Pause for muscle memory retention.

Inhale toward your lower back and side ribs, and feel your spine lengthen. Exhale, and slowly move your shoulders downward as low as possible. Feel your collarbones widen, your shoulder blades flatten, your lat muscles connect with your core abdominals, and your whole-body muscle connection engage from your feet to your head. Maintain the length of your spine as it slowly returns to the anchoring position.

Repetitions: Three.

Variations: Forehead on knees. Anchoring Position.

Advanced: Lie on mat supine with knees bent, feet standing; supine with legs extended; prone with legs extended.

POSITION 2

Anchoring Position is the same as beginning use.

With less rounding than the beginning use, place the cervical, thoracic, and lumbar areas of your spine in a smooth, even curve. Lead with the top of your sternum to lean slightly forward. Inhale toward your lower back and side ribs. Feel your shoulder blades slide back and down your ribs.

Exhale, and slowly roll your shoulders forward into armored "protect the heart" position. Relax muscle tension of other areas.

Pause for muscle memory retention.

Inhale toward your lower back and side ribs. Maintain your sternum positioned forward and upward. Exhale, and slowly broaden your shoulders away from protective posture and into balanced, alpha shoulder alignment. Your body is ready for activity rather than protection when you feel your collarbones widen, shoulder blades flatten, your lat muscles connect with your core abdominal muscles, and your whole body muscle connection engage from your feet to your head.

Repetitions: Three.

 POSITION 3

Anchoring Position is the same as beginning use, with less rounding. Place the cervical, thoracic, and lumbar areas of your spine in a smooth, even curve. Chin Lifts are useful to develop this alignment.

Place your toes together and upward, heels apart with your ankles reaching inward and your elbows outward. Broaden your shoulders by reaching the top of your sternum forward and up with your lower end back and down to activate core abdominals, evidenced by a hollow below your anterior ribs. Imagine drawing a square with the shoulders. Slowly reach your shoulders forward, and then slowly lift the shoulders upward.

Pause for muscle memory retention.

Maintain your elbows outward and the top of your sternum forward and up. Slowly reach your shoulders back, and feel muscles bring your shoulder blades close to the spine.

Slowly move your shoulders down toward your back jean pockets and outward. Feel all the surface and core muscles of your shoulder girdle, pelvic girdle, and arms, the hollows in your armpits, and your abdominal area.

Repetitions: Three.

Arm Exercises—Triangle 4

Objectives: To balance strength and flexibility between muscles in the front and back of your arms and shoulders. Shoulder muscles attach to your upper nine ribs, neck, and head. Shoulders require the anchoring of core and surface muscles in these areas and the lumbar spine to support and securely stabilize your shoulder joints while your arms are in motion.

Anchoring Position: Lie supine on a mat with your knees bent, feet standing parallel at right angles to foreleg, toes lifted, heels separated with Achilles tendons behind the space between toes two and three. Place your knees, great toes, and toe joints together. Lift the lateral borders of your feet to place your ankles toward the midline and balance weight over the arches between your great, second, and third toes and the inner half of your heel. Feel your core inner thigh and core lower back abdominal muscles.

Position your pelvis in neutral with your waistline rolled back and your SI joint dimples and the L1-T12 apex of Triangles 3 and 4 flat on the mat to lengthen and balance your lumbar curve. Reach your sit bones toward your feet, with the top of your breastbone toward the ceiling and your head. Reach the lower part of your breastbone toward the mat and your feet. With both ends of your lumbar curve anchored (SI joint dimples and L1-T12 apex), your body is secure for movement. Feel your hips narrow and your core abdominal muscles create a deeper hollow below your front ribs.

Your shoulder position has wide collarbones, with your shoulder blades back and down toward your back jean pockets and your sternum horizontal, as described above. Feel your core shoulder muscles and the hollow below your front ribs. With your chin toward the sternum and the backs of your ears and crown of your head reaching away from your shoulders, you should feel your facial muscles activated, naturally lifting any sagging facial muscles.

Arm Rotations

 POSITION 1

Anchoring Position: Arms diagonal, palms down, middle fingers in line with the midline of your wrists and elbows, and thumbs straight in a right angle position from your fingers to activate core muscles of your shoulder girdle and place your shoulder blades inward. Reach your knees away from your head to roll your waist back into a pelvic tilt. Close your eyes, and slowly move your arms to the position where they feel shoulder level. Open your eyes, and see where you felt your arms were placed. Often, where we feel our body parts are positioned may not be where they actually are. Reposition your arms if necessary *(fig. 30).*

Lift your arms slightly above the mat. Lock your elbows, and feel the surface muscles of your arms, shoulders, and chest activated. Unlock your elbows, and feel the core muscles of your shoulder joint engaged. With tense protective surface muscles relaxed, core muscles are able to stabilize your shoulder joint while surface muscles move your arms.

Slowly lift your arms up toward the ceiling with your palms facing outward. Place the backs of your hands and fingers together, reaching toward the ceiling, thumbs at a right angle, straight and touching. To find the vertical light line of gravity for the arms and hands, explore. Notice

FIGURE 30

arm rotations

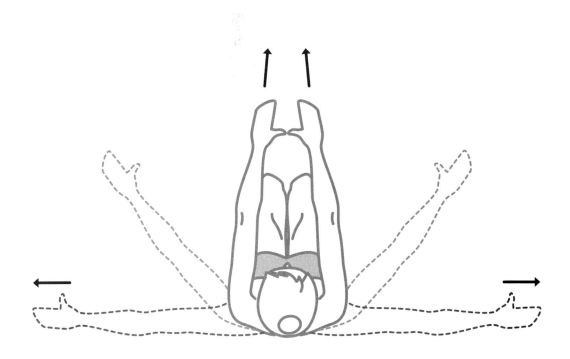

when your arms begin to feel heavy when you slowly sway them in small movements forward and backward. Then find the place where they feel the lightest. Maintain your thumbs in a straight line. If your thumbs are not straight, your thumb muscles are hyperextended and weak and your thumb joints are compressed. This is the joint where arthritis first occurs.

Pause for muscle memory retention.

Retain lengthening of your spine with your chin toward your breastbone, the backs of your ears reaching away from your shoulders, shoulders reaching toward your hips, the L1-T12 apex anchored, and your knees reaching away from your head. Feel the light line of gravity, and slowly begin to lower your arms to the right-angle beginning position. As your arms move away from the vertical line of gravity, feel how much the weight of your arms increases as they get closer to the floor. Pause before your palms touch the floor. Reach your shoulders outward, and feel the activation of many core and surface muscles broaden your shoulders, support your shoulder joints, and lighten your load. Lower your palms to the floor.

Repetitions: One for Positions 1, 2, 3, and 4.

Ⓑ POSITION 2

Anchoring Position is the same as Arm Rotations from Position 1. Raise your arms slightly above the floor to turn your hands and position your thumbs toward the ceiling. Lower the hands, placing the little finger side of your hands and wrists on the floor, with a straight line from your middle fingers through your wrists to your elbows. Reach your knees away from your head to lengthen the front of your hips and roll your waist back to the mat into a pelvic tilt position. Release tension in your shoulders, and slide your shoulder blades toward your back jean pockets.

Inhale toward your lower back and side ribs. Exhale, and slowly lift your arms upward. Maintain the elbows turned outward as your thumbs come together at a right angle to your fingers as they lift toward the ceiling, creating a goal-post position with your hands.

Pause for muscle memory retention.

With your elbows turned outward, feel your triceps and lat muscles engaged. Inhale toward your lower back and side ribs to anchor the L1-T12 apex. Exhale, reach your shoulders outward, and lead with your elbows to slowly lower your arms toward the floor. Pause before your arms touch the floor. Add more muscle energy, reaching outward with the shoulders. Feel the support of the core muscles at your shoulder joints. Lower the little finger side of your hands and wrists to the floor.

POSITION 3

Anchoring Position is the same as Arm Rotations from Position 1. Raise your arms above the floor, turn your palms upward, and lower the back of your hands to the floor with your thumbs at a right angle. Feel your little fingers and thumbs on the floor.

Inhale toward your lower back and side ribs to anchor the L1-T12 apex. Reach your knees away from your head to lengthen the front of your hips; maintain your pelvic tilt. Exhale, and slowly lift your arms upward, your elbows pointing outward and your palms facing inward. When your palms come together, reach your fingers toward the ceiling and your thumbs away from your fingers. Lengthen your arms with your elbows pointing outward. Feel the engagement of your triceps and lat muscles. Feel how you lose these muscles in action if your elbows are not turned outward.

Pause for muscle memory retention.

Inhale toward your lower back and side ribs. Ease your shoulders back and down toward your back jean pockets and your chin toward your sternum with the back of your neck long. Exhale. Maintain your palms facing inward, and lead with your elbows to slowly lower your arms toward the floor. Before they reach the floor, pause and reach your shoulders outward to activate additional core shoulder joint muscles. Lower your arms. Your elbows will reach the floor slightly before the backs of your hands.

(B) POSITION 4

Anchoring Position is the same as Arm Rotations from Position 1. Reach your knees away from your hips and the backs of your ears away from your shoulders to stabilize your lengthened spine and maintain your pelvic tilt. Lift your arms. Rotate them one quarter turn, placing your thumbs on the floor and the little finger side of your hands toward the ceiling. Feel your collarbones widen and your shoulder blades drawn closer together.

Inhale toward your lower back and side ribs to anchor the L1-T12 apex. Exhale. Reach your fingertips outward and slowly lift your arms upward to bring the little finger sides of your hands together like an open book.

Pause for muscle memory retention.

Reach your shoulders back and down toward your back jean pockets, the backs of your ears away from your shoulders and your knees away from your head, with your spine lengthened from both ends. Inhale toward your lower back and side ribs. Maintain the little finger side of your hands upward. Exhale, and slowly lower your arms toward the floor. When your thumbs touch the floor, anchor your collarbones wide and your shoulders broad. Turn your palms upward, and rest the back of your hands on the floor. Return your pelvis to neutral.

Variation: Reverse the sequence, beginning with Position 4-1, and turn your hands before they return to the floor.

Anchoring Position Options: Anchoring Position Standing to strengthen deltoid muscles. Here's a personal example: My first college major was in music and piano performance. My elbows were always below my shoulders, and my deltoid muscles were rarely used. After graduation, while teaching elementary music, my first experience writing on the chalkboard was painful. My shoulder joint had bursitis, irritation of the bursa of my shoulder joint, from weak deltoid support.

Practicing these Dailey Inner Core Workout arm and shoulder movements will maintain deltoid muscle strength so that you may easily reach for something at shoulder level or above without discomfort in your shoulder joint.

Circle Arm Movements

Objectives: To balance strength and flexibility between the muscles of your arms, shoulders, neck, upper torso, and spine. Your arms and shoulders require anchoring of core and surface muscles in these areas to support and stabilize your shoulder joints while your arms move in lateral circular movements outward from the hips to shoulder level and upward toward the head.

Anchoring Position: Supine or Prone. For beginning movements, lie supine on a mat with your knees bent, your feet standing parallel at a right angle to your foreleg, your toes lifted, and your heels separated, with the Achilles tendon behind the space between toes two and three. Place your knees, great toes, and toe joints together, the lateral borders of your feet lifted to reach your ankles toward the midline, and balance the weight over your arches between the great, second, and third toes and inner half of your heel. Feel your core inner thigh, lower back, and abdominal muscles.

Position your pelvis in neutral, your waistline rolled back with both ends of your lumbar curve, SI joint dimples, and the L1-T12 apex anchored to the mat and your sit bones reaching toward your feet to lengthen your spine and narrow your hips. To flatten your shoulder blades onto the mat, widen your collarbones and reach your shoulder blades back toward the mat and down toward your back jean pockets, with the upper end of your sternum toward the ceiling and your head, the lower end of your sternum toward the mat and your feet.

Place your arms long beside your thighs, palms down, middle fingers in line with the midline of your wrists and elbows, thumbs straight and pointing toward your thighs in a right angle position to your fingers, and your elbows pointing outward with elbow windows open. Notice if your elbows, wrists, and hands of both arms are on the mat. If not, are your heels apart, ankles inward, knees together, hips narrowed, and spine lengthened? Eventually, when all triangles are aligned through Dailey Inner Core Workout movements, even the smallest of muscle imbalance areas will be fixed.

Inhale toward your lower back and side ribs to anchor the L1-T12 apex. Reach your knees away from your head to lengthen the front of your hips, and roll your waist back into a pelvic tilt to lengthen your spine and narrow your hips.

(B) QUARTER CIRCLE ARM MOVEMENTS

Press your shoulder blades back flat onto the mat, and feel rhomboid muscles squeeze your shoulder blades toward the spine *(fig. 31)*. Notice that the lower tips of your shoulder blades point down and inward toward your waist. Exhale. With your arms long, lead with your elbows and slowly slide your arms outward and upward into a diagonal position. Notice that your rhomboid muscles are still squeezing your shoulder blades toward your spine. Slowly slide your

FIGURE 31

quarter circle arm movements

This exercise can be done standing, laying down on your back, or laying down with legs bent. Keep shoulders back and down.

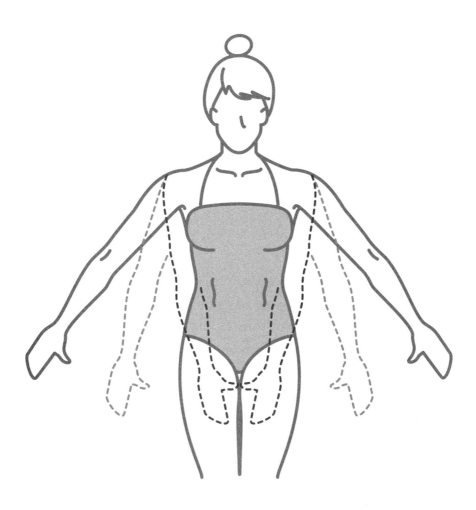

arms upward to shoulder level, and feel the lower tip of your shoulder blades slide outward away from your spine and upward to allow your arms to move into shoulder level position.

Pause for muscle memory retention.

Notice that your collarbones have remained wide. Inhale toward your lower back and side ribs. Maintain long arms and unlocked elbows. Reach your shoulders out toward your elbows, and feel more inner core muscles activated at your shoulder joints and armpits. Exhale. Anchor the L1-T12 apex and shoulders back toward the mat. Slowly slide your arms downward with core muscle action. Feel lower- and middle-trapezius muscles move the lower tip of your shoulder blades downward and inward until they are squeezed toward the spine by your rhomboid muscles. The arms have returned to the diagonal arm position.

Repetitions: One.

Options: Anchoring Position Standing and Supine with legs extended.

 HALF CIRCLE ARM MOVEMENTS
Separate your heels, and reach your ankles inward with your toes lifted and arms shoulder level, palms down, fingers softly together, your middle fingers in line with the midline of your wrists, with elbows and thumbs straight to form a right angle with your fingers *(fig. 32)*. Reach your knees away from your head, and roll your waist back into a pelvic tilt. Feel your core abdominal and knee fist muscles. Inhale, and feel your lower back lengthen and side ribs widen. Reinforce your shoulder blades back and down toward your back jean pockets with your elbows pointing outward. Exhale, and slowly slide your arms down beside your thighs. Leading with your thumbs, slowly trace your palms over your thighs until your thumbs come together in the goalpost position.

FIGURE 32
half circle arm movements

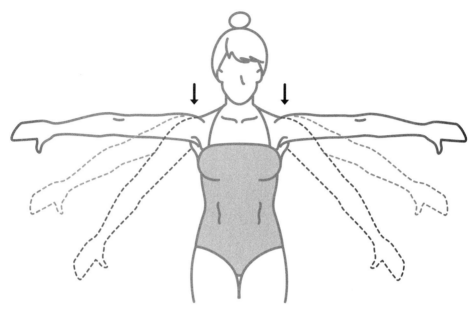

FIRST QUARTER

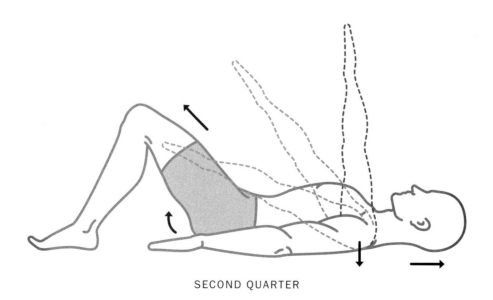

SECOND QUARTER

Widen your shoulders to activate additional core and surface muscles. Lead with your elbows to lift your arms upward, placing your arms and hands into a vertical line above your collarbones.

Pause for muscle memory retention.

Reach your shoulders outward. Feel a squeeze inside your armpits and shoulder joints as your core muscles broaden, and anchor your shoulder blades back toward the mat and down toward your hips. Inhale toward your lower back and side ribs. Reach your knees away from your hips to anchor your pelvis and lengthen your spine. Exhale, and, with your elbows pointing outward and shoulders anchored, lengthen your arms upward and slowly move the arms outward, placing the little finger side of your hands at shoulder level near the floor. Maintain your shoulders, reaching wide and down toward your hips as your elbows turn the forearm and palms downward, and place your hands and elbows on the floor.

Repetitions: One.

Options: Anchoring Position Standing and Supine with legs extended.

 WHOLE CIRCLE ARM MOVEMENTS

Anchoring Position: Prone, with your great toes and knees together. Press your pubic bone downward. Reach your sit bones pointed toward your heels and the L1-T12 apex toward the ceiling *(fig. 33)*. Feel gluteal muscles activate and hips narrow with your pelvis in prone, neutral position. Relax your toes. Point and tilt your feet inward, placing your outer borders and little toes on the mat—the opposite of supine position. Maintain your heels apart as your ankles reach inward. Rest your forehead on the mat with your shoulders broad, hands with arms long beside your thighs, elbows

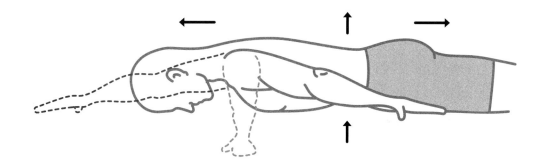

FIGURE 33

whole circle arm movements

Keep sit bones pointed toward your feet so you have a balanced curve at the back of the waist.

unlocked, and palms of hands flat on the mat with your fingers softly together, middle fingers in line with the midline of your wrists and elbows, and thumbs straight at a right angle to your hands.

Gently press your forehead into the mat; anchor your pelvis to secure your lumbar spine and midline of support. Reach your shoulders toward the ceiling, down toward back jean pockets, and outward to activate core and surface shoulder muscles. Slowly move your arms in a long line from the shoulders through the elbows, wrists, and middle fingers to shoulder level. Maintain your collarbones wide, shoulder blades flat against your ribs, and elbows pointed upward. Feel active core and surface shoulder blade and shoulder joint muscles. Slowly continue. Notice that your collarbone and shoulder blade core muscles initiate the muscle action to slide your arms upward and bring your thumbs into the goal post position above your head.

Pause for muscle memory retention.

Reinforce all of the above Anchoring Position muscles, and maintain stabilization of your feet, legs, spine, and elbows, pointing upward as your collarbones and shoulder blades slowly move your arms downward and replacing your hands beside your thighs.

Repetitions: One.

Option: Half Circle Arm Movements into Whole Circle Arm Movements. In supine position, after your arms slide to shoulder level with your palms downward, maintain the length of your arms and continue sliding your arms upward with your palms down. When they come to their highest point, turn your palms upward with your thumbs and fingers on the floor. Continue to slowly slide your arms up until your thumbs come together. Pause, reinforce, and return your arms downward as you had moved them upward.

Forward & Backward Sways

Objectives: To take the body to standing erect position, utilizing balanced and strengthened core and surface muscles developed by Dailey Inner Core Workout movements executed in the supine position. Sways have a strong influence on creating balance between the body's anterior and posterior muscle strength. The process also includes a reset of the inner ear balance sensor (vestibular apparatus) and its communication with proprioceptors. These movements are like the body's very own Global Positioning System. Practicing the movements will "reroute" dysfunctional, non-erect posture to a natural, erect, and balanced standing posture.

Anchoring Position: Stand with your toes together, heels apart, and Achilles tendon behind the space between toes two and three, placing your feet in parallel alignment *(fig. 34)*. This foot placement gives your body a rectangular base of support that is more stable than a triangular base, in which the heels are together. Place knees together unlocked and at the ready. Tilt your pelvis and hip points (ASIS) backward, pubic bone forward, and sit bones pointed toward your heels, with narrowed hips and your pelvis in neutral. Reach the low end of your sternum back and down to anchor the L5-T12 apex, with the upper end of your sternum forward and up to broaden your shoulders. Lengthen your cervical spine, level your head, and place your arms centered in a vertical line with your hips, knees, and ankles.

Reach your ankles inward; keep your shoulders wide as your elbows reach outward to open your elbow windows, increase your respiratory capacity, and tone your triceps. Turn your toes up, close your eyes, and feel the oscillation of your body as your inner-ear balance sensor (the vestibule of the ear) communicates to the brain how to find the centerline of gravity without assistance from your eyes. Do you have more body weight on the forefeet or heels, or is your weight balanced and centered over the arches of your feet?

With your eyes open, maintain standing alignment and sway your body forward from your ankles, placing weight on your inner three metatarsals (ball of your foot bones). This allows the anterior surface muscles from your feet to your head to relax and your inner core muscles to participate in erect vertical posture. It also gives an extreme example of information, transmitted from proprioceptors of the feet into the inner ear, about your body's alignment positioned away from your central line of gravity. Maintain narrowed hips, your pelvis in neutral with your pubic bone forward, sit bones reaching toward your heels, and your shoulders broad with length at the back of your neck and waist. Reach your knees away from your head, and feel muscle activation of your knee fist, inner thigh, and inner core low abdominal muscles continuing through to your head.

Pause for muscle memory retention.

Reinforce your toes upward, ankles inward, hips narrow, pelvis in neutral position, shoulders broad, and the back of your neck and waist long with your elbows turned outward. Sway your body back toward your heels, and notice the feel of passing through the central line of gravity. The posterior surface muscles relax and your inner core muscles become active, balanced partners with your anterior muscles.

Return to erect standing position.

Repetitions: Three.

Following the third repetition, keep your toes lifted, close your eyes, and feel the decrease in oscillation of your body. The improved sense of your body being able to find its true center of balance and support is an indication that stronger inner ear and proprioceptive functions have improved in your feet and all areas of your body.

FIGURE 34

forward and backward sways

Keep shoulders back and down.

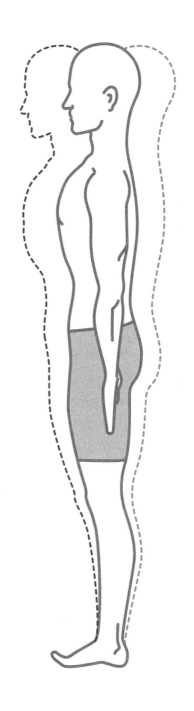

Forward Bends

Objectives: To balance structural support of your anterior and posterior surfaces and inner core muscles between both ends of the spine initiated from the standing position.

Anchoring Position: Standing with your toes together, heels apart, and Achilles tendon behind the space between toes two and three, place your feet in parallel alignment to provide your body a sense of balance with a rectangular base of support. Position your knees together, unlocked and at the ready, with your pelvis and hip points (ASIS) tilted back, pubic bone forward, and sit bones reaching toward your heels with your hips narrowed and your pelvis in neutral. Reach the low end of your sternum back and down, toward your feet, to anchor your L1-T12 apex and the upper end of your sternum forward and up, toward your head, to broaden your shoulders, lengthen your cervical spine, and level your head; place your arms centered in a vertical line with your hips, knees, and ankles.

(B) ROUND BEND

Tilt your feet inward to lift your outer arches, and turn your toes upward with your chin toward your sternum and the backs of your ears reaching away from your shoulders to maintain length in the upper end of your spine *(fig. 35)*. Reach your knees away from your head to increase your core knee fist, inner thigh, hip-narrowing, and low abdominal muscles. Maintain your lengthened lower end of the spine with your pelvis in neutral. Both ends of your spine must be anchored in order to activate the core muscles that surround all of your vertebrae.

Maintain the length in the front of your hips and your pelvis in neutral position, with your chin toward your sternum, the backs of your ears reaching away from your

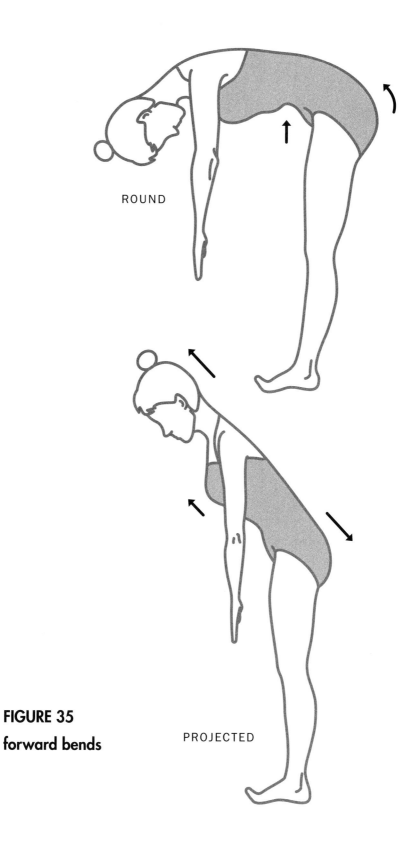

ROUND

PROJECTED

FIGURE 35
forward bends

167

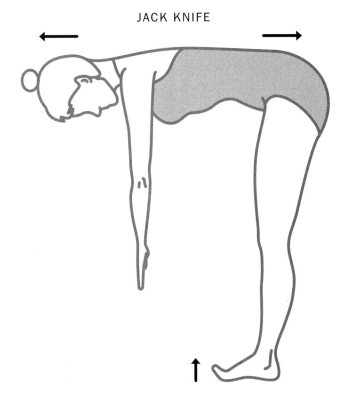

JACK KNIFE

FIGURE 35
forward bends

shoulders, and your sit bones pointed toward your heels and balanced over the arches of your feet. Lead with your forehead, and, with an equal movement at each vertebra, bend your spine forward from the base of the skull downward to the first lumbar vertebra connected to your sacrum. There is a tendency to bend at the hips, the seventh cervical vertebra, and between the shoulder blades. Be aware of these areas as you practice the Round Bend in order to move correctly and gain the benefits. Excess bends at C7, the hips, and shoulders will weaken all abdominal muscle layers.

Pause for muscle memory retention.

Maintain your toes lifted, and stabilize your pelvis with your sit bones pointed toward your heels and your pubic bone forward. Feel your core abdominal hollow, narrowed hips, and the back of your neck long. With your collarbones wide, your shoulders broad, the back of your neck reaching away from the floor, your arms long in a vertical line from your shoulders, and your elbows turned outward, feel the connection between your triceps and shoulder girdle muscles, along with toned core abdominal muscles. With the pelvis anchored, lead with the back of your neck and upper end of your sternum to slowly return, vertebra by vertebra, to a balanced, standing alignment. When reaching the upright standing position, lift your ribs up out of your hips and the backs of your ears upward and away from your shoulders. Feel lengthening of your spine, narrowing of your hips, and broadening of your shoulders. Notice your toned and lifted gluteal and facial muscles.

Repetitions: One.

Variation 1: Projected Bend your spine forward from the hips into a diagonal line while maintaining a lengthened spine, narrowed hips, and broad shoulders (*fig. 35*).

(A) *Variation 2: Jack Knife* Bend the spine forward from the hips, placing your spine into a horizontal, tabletop position *(fig. 35)*.

Option: Anchoring Position Sitting on a chair or mat.

(B) FORWARD BEND KNEELING

(I) *Objectives:* To create a balance of surface and core muscles between the anterior and posterior sides of your spine and correct irregular lumbar curvatures.

Anchoring Position: Kneeling on a mat, place your knees and toe joints together, ankles reaching inward with outer borders of your feet and little toes on the mat *(fig. 36)*. Tilt your pubic bone upward, with your hip points back and sit bones toward the back of your knees, to lengthen the front of your hips, lengthen your lumbar curve, and narrow your hips. Notice the challenge of achieving erect alignment and anchoring the pelvis in neutral when the foundation of support is on your knees rather than your feet. Standing gives your knees freedom to hyperextend, hip flexors to tighten, and pelvis to tilt forward, shortening your lumbar curve and broadening your hips.

With elbows bent, place hands lightly on a bench or chair, your collarbones wide and shoulder blades down toward back jean pockets. In one unit from your tailbone to your head, bend the spine forward from your hips into a diagonal line. Maintain your hips over your knees, a light touch of your hands on the bench, shoulders broad with the backs of your ears reaching away from your shoulders, and your sit bones reaching away from your head to lengthen your spine. Reach your knees into mat. Feel your core-anchoring muscles from your knee joints to your pelvis. Tip your pubic bone upward into a pelvic tilt to lengthen the front of your hips and lumbar spine in order to strengthen your core abdominals.

Pause for muscle memory retention.

With a small sway of your hips back toward your heels, add more tilt to your pelvis and length to the back of your waist. Feel a stretch in front of your hips, toned gluteals, and deep, core abdominal hollow muscles. Maintain your broad shoulders and long neck. After three repetitions of small sways forward and backward, maintain the increased length at the back of your waist, reach your knees into the mat, and lead with the back of your neck and top of sternum to return to upright Anchoring Position.

Repetitions: Three.

Rotational Movements

Objectives: To balance strength and flexibility between the surface and inner core muscles that allow your head and spine to rotate separately to the right and to the left.

Anchoring Position: Sit on chair with your knees bent and feet standing in Triangle 1 position, with your toes up and ankles reaching inward *(fig. 37)*.

Alternate Anchoring Position: Sit on a mat with the soles of your feet together and knees open into a diamond shape, with your feet the length of your forearm from your pelvis. Place your chin toward your sternum, head level, wrists on your knees with palms upward, elbows outward, and collar-bones wide to maintain your broad shoulders.

ROTATIONAL MOVEMENTS OF THE HEAD

Turn your toes upward. Feel your pelvis centered over your sit bones and your inner core abdominal muscles activated. Lift your ribs upward from your hips and the backs of your ears upward from your shoulders. Anchor the L1-T12 apex, and feel your lengthened lumbar and cervical spine.

FIGURE 36

forward bends: kneeling

Keep the opening of the ear vertical with the elbows out. Keep shoulders wide and reaching away from your ears.

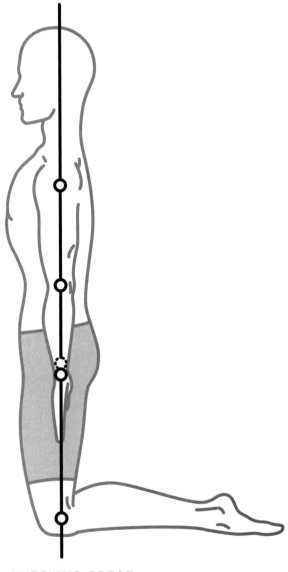

KNEELING ERECT

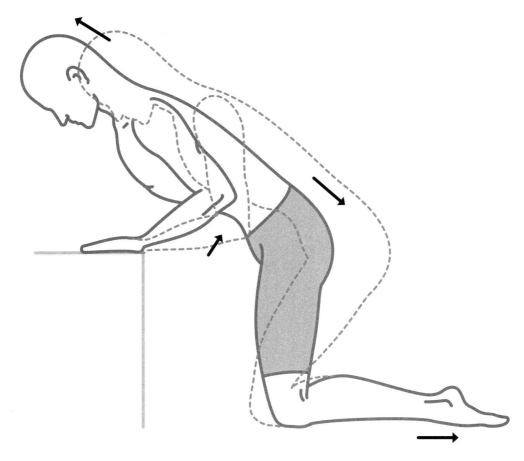

PROJECTED TO SITTING TOWARDS HEELS

173

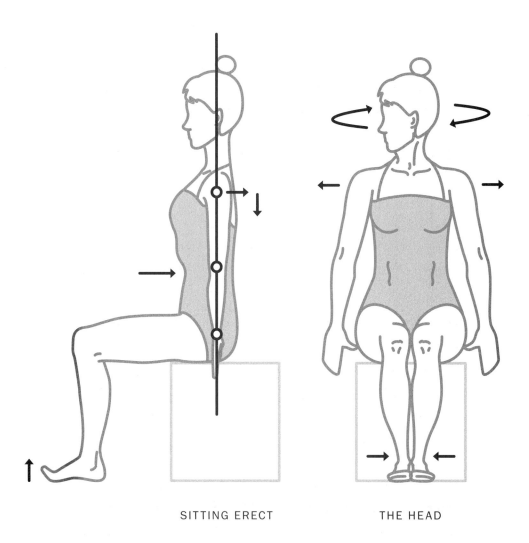

SITTING ERECT   THE HEAD

FIGURE 37

rotational movements

Keep toes up, elbows out, ankles in, and shoulders wide.

174

Inhale toward your lower back and side ribs. With your head level and your chin toward your sternum, exhale; with core neck muscles, slowly rotate your head to the right. Feel when activation begins at the sternocleidomastoid muscle, which is attached to the skull behind the left ear and ends at the sternum. When your left ear is in line with your sternum, this long surface muscle is placed in the mid-vertical line along with your sternum and spine.

Pause for muscle memory retention.

Reinforce your ribs upward from the hips. Inhale toward your lower back and side ribs. Lift the backs of your ears upward to maintain length in your cervical spine. Exhale, and notice when the surface sternocleidomastoid muscle begins to relax as your core neck muscles slowly rotate your head to face forward with your chin toward your sternum and your head level. Repeat the head rotation to the left.

Repetitions: Three. Rotation distance increases with each repetition.

Option: Before rotating your head, turn your eyes to the right, return forward, and repeat the eye turn to the left. Follow with your eyes leading before each head rotation. Notice a major increase in the distance of rotation when your eyes lead.

In another interesting eye connection, the equestrian teacher of one of my students told her that movement of the eyes has an inner connection to the rider's hips and thighs. When riding a horse that is leaping over a jump and about to land, without pulling on the reins, turn your eyes in the direction you want it to go. Sitting with your hips on the saddle, the horse will receive a feeling from your eyes to your right or left hip and follow the command.

When your head is facing forward, the right and left sternocleidomastoid muscles normally are in a balanced resting state and unnoticeable. However, one of my former students had both protruding at the same time. I had never seen the muscles visible when a face was forward. Later that day, I imitated the student's forward head alignment and was shocked at how tight my cranial muscles were. Years later, after reading the book *Cancer is Not a Disease*, I realized how much tension the student's body must have been carrying, which therefore was blocking oxygen to her body systems. Later, I learned this former student had died from cancer.

ROTATIONAL MOVEMENTS OF THE SPINE AND HEAD

Turn your toes upward. Feel your pelvis centered over your sit bones and inner core abdominal muscles activated.

Place your hands on your shoulders, fingers in front and thumbs back, with your elbows at shoulder level and reaching outward. Lift your ribs up out of your hips and the backs of your ears upward from your shoulders. Inhale toward your lower back and side ribs. Anchor the L1-T12 apex, and feel your lengthened lumbar and cervical spine. Exhale, and, in sequence, slowly turn your eyes to the right, followed by your face, shoulders, and ribs.

Pause for muscle memory retention.

With your elbows wide, inhale directly toward your right lung. Reinforce your ribs, and, with the backs of your ears lifted, slowly in sequence rotate forward your ribs and shoulders, face, and eyes forward. Repeat the rotation of your spine to the left, and direct inhalation toward your left lung.

Notice if rotation is easier on one side than the other. If so, right- or left-handed habits may cause more tense muscles on the dominant side.

Repetitions: Three, and follow with a Sitting Forward Bend.

Lateral Bends

Objectives: To balance strength and flexibility between surface and inner core muscles on the right and left sides of the neck and waist, lift weight of body up from the atlas (first) cervical and from the fifth (lowest) lumbar vertebrae, provide strong foundations for the head and shoulder girdle, and release tension and pain in the neck and lower back.

Anchoring Position: Sit on a mat with soles of your feet together, knees open in a diamond shape, with your feet the length of your forearm from your pelvis, chin toward your sternum, the backs of your ears reaching up away from your shoulders, wrists on your knees with palms upward, elbows outward, and your collarbones wide to maintain broad shoulders.

LATERAL BENDS OF THE HEAD

With your big toe metatarsals and inner edge of your heels together, turn your toes upward, and lift your heels *(fig. 38)*. Lift your ribs up away from your hips and the backs of your ears up away from your shoulders. Anchor the L1-T12 apex. Feel your lengthened lumbar and cervical spine.

Inhale toward your lower back and side ribs. Maintain your neck long and nose in alignment with your sternum. Exhale, and place your hands on your shoulders, thumbs at your collarbones and two fingers on the side of your neck at jaw level in order to move your head separately from your neck at the atlas vertebra. Tilt your head to the right as your chin moves like a windshield wiper to the left. Feel the right sternocleidomastoid muscle.

Pause for muscle memory retention.

Inhale toward your lower back and side ribs. Anchor your shoulders backward, outward, and downward, toward your back jean pockets. Exhale, and return your head to level with your windshield-wiper chin down toward your sternum and the backs of your ears lifting up away from your shoulders. Repeat on your left side, and follow with a Sitting Forward Bend.

Repetitions: Three.

LATERAL BENDS OF THE TRUNK AND HEAD

Dominant hand use increases the lateral curve at the waist on the right side for right-handers and left side for left-handers *(fig. 38)*. With an increase in the lateral curve, the shoulder and fingers are usually lower on the dominant side.

To begin the lateral movements to help improve the curvatures, place your big toe metatarsals and the inner edge of your heels together, turn your toes upward, and lift your heels. Place your hands on your shoulders, your thumbs at your collarbones, and your fingers on your head beside your ears with elbows and shoulders reaching outward. Lift your ribs upward from your hips and the backs of your ears upward from your shoulders. Anchor L1-T12, and feel your lengthened lumbar and cervical spine. Inhale toward your lower back and side ribs. Imagine a fist between your right ribs and hip. Exhale. Maintain the space between your ribs and hip, anchor your left sit bone toward the mat, and bend your ribs, shoulders, neck, and head together into a curve toward the right.

Pause for muscle memory retention.

Inhale toward your left lung. Maintain space between your right ribs and hip, with your shoulders broad and your ribs, shoulders, neck, and head working together as one unit. With both sit bones anchored to the mat, return to the upright position; lift your ribs up away from your hips and the backs of your ears up away from your shoulders. Repeat on the left side. Notice if there is less flexibility when the bend is away from your dominant side.

Repetitions: Three, and follow with a Forward Bend.

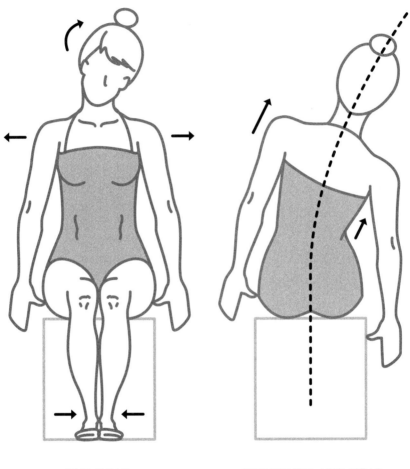

THE HEAD   THE TRUNK AND HEAD

FIGURE 38

lateral bends

Keep nose directly above space between collar bone and keep as much space between your right ribs and hip as you tilt to the right.

Knee Bends

Objectives: To take development of balanced inner core and surface muscles of all six triangles into the upright position. The goal is for your balanced surface and core muscles to have the ability to place the base lines of Triangles 2, 3, 4, and 5 and the apex of Triangles 3 and 4 against the wall.

Anchoring Position: Stand with back of your pelvis and shoulders against a wall with your heels approximately one inch from the baseboard *(fig. 39).* Place your feet parallel with your toes together, heels apart, and Achilles tendon behind the center of your forefoot, with your knees together and un-locked, head level, arms long beside thighs, and your elbows pointing outward with your elbow windows open.

Movement: Tilt your feet inward, and turn your toes upward. Notice what parts of the posterior side of the pelvis, verte-brae, and shoulders are against the wall. Are the SI joint dim-ples of your pelvis against the wall? Slowly bend your knees, and slide down a few inches. Tilt your pelvis back toward the wall with your pubic bone forward and sit bones pointed toward your heels. Feel your core low abdominal muscles kick in and SI joint dimples (the low anchor of your lumbar curve) against the wall. Are the vertebrae behind your ster-num and shoulder blades flat against the wall? Reach the low end of your sternum back toward the wall and down toward your heels to anchor the upper end of your lumbar curve, the L1-T12 apex. Reach the top end of your sternum forward and upward, away from the low end of your sternum, to assist your shoulder blades and all of the thoracic vertebrae above T12 to feel the wall.

Place your head in a comfortable, level position with your neck long and the back of your head near the wall. Rarely is the head able to touch the wall when it is level and centered during the Knee Bend experience. With continued practice

FIGURE 39
knee bends

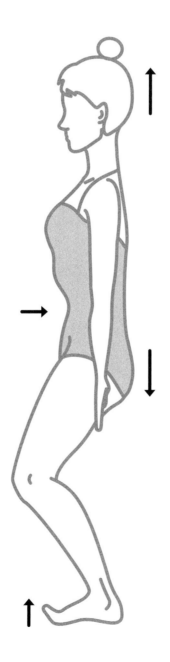

of Dailey Inner Core Workout movements, your head will be able to reach the wall with your neck long and your head level and centered above your shoulders and spine.

Pause for muscle memory retention.

With your heels apart, ankles inward, and toes lifted, reach your knees away from your head to activate your inner knee fist and abdominal muscles. Slowly lengthen your knees to standing position. Feel your knee stabilization, inner thigh, hip-narrowing, abdominal-hollow, and core muscles connecting through to your head. Maintain unlocked knees, narrowed hips, length at the back of your waist and neck, broad shoulders, elbows turned outward, and head balanced and centered, with the backs of your ears reaching upwardward away from your shoulders.

Repetitions: Three.

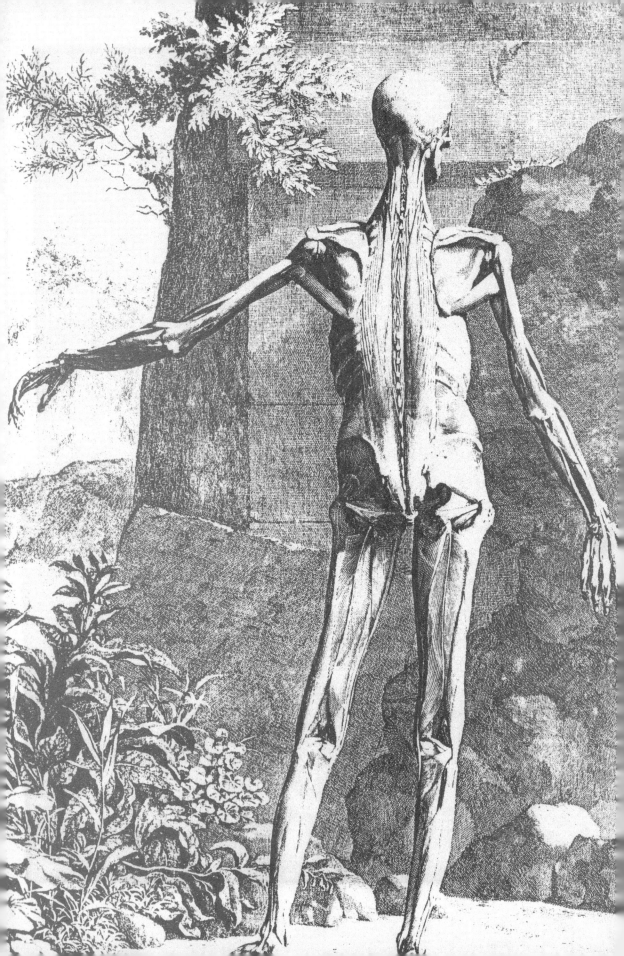

PART THREE

LESSON PLANS

"STRENGTH AND FLEXIBILITY OF THE CORE MUSCLES DETERMINE
THE SHAPE OF OUTER MUSCLES AND THE ENTIRE BODY."

—ALICE ANN DAILEY

DAILEY INNER CORE WORKOUT LESSON PLANS

Now that you know all of the moves of the Dailey Inner Body Workout, you will be able to combine them to create an effective workout. Eight different plans that each take about thirty minutes to execute are provided, starting with the beginning movements and progressing to the intermediate and advanced movements. Plan 1 is a beginning plan. Over time, as your body becomes more familiar with the movements, you may execute them sequentially and progress as you master each plan. Even when you have gained the ability to perform the advanced movements, it is still important to practice the beginning and intermediate movements in order to maintain strength in all of your inner core muscles.

PLAN 1

① **Knee Bends** *Fig. 39   p. 181*

② **Foot Movements** *Fig. 18   p. 104*

③ **Leg Rotations** *Fig. 20   p. 112*

④ **Shoulder Movements** *Fig. 29   p. 146*

⑤ **Pelvic Tilt** *Fig. 24   p. 127*

⑥ **Medium Pelvic Lift** *Fig. 24   p. 127*

⑦ **High Head Lift** *Fig. 25   p. 132*

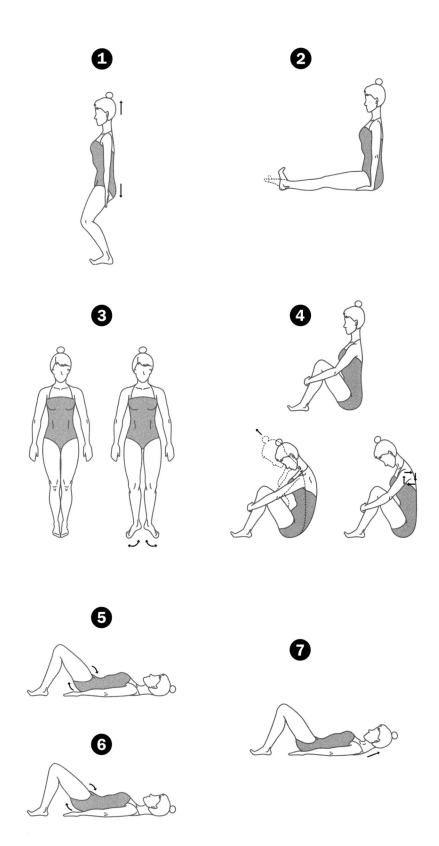

187

PLAN 2

(1) **Forward & Backward Sways**   *Fig. 34   p. 165*

(2) **Forward Bends**   *Fig. 36   p. 172–73*

(3) **Pelvic Tilt**   *Fig. 24   p. 127*

(4) **Low to Medium Chin Lift**   *Fig. 26   p. 136*

(5) **Narrow Knee Spread**   *Fig. 22   p. 122*

(6) **Medium Pelvic Lift**   *Fig. 24   p. 127*

(7) **High Head Lift**   *Fig. 25   p. 132*

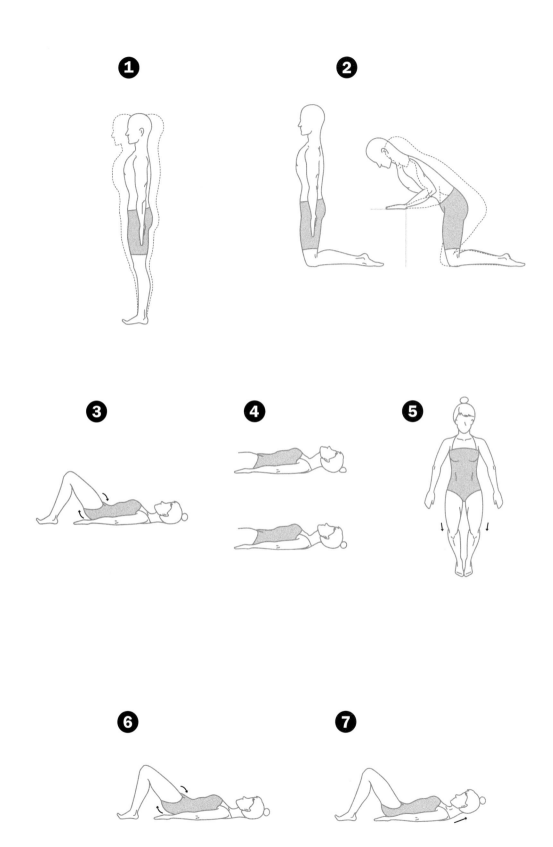

189

PLAN 3

① Low to Medium Chin Lift   *Fig. 26   p. 136*

② Forward Bends   *Fig. 35   p. 167–68*

③ Narrow to Medium Knee Spread   *Fig. 22   p. 122*

④ Medium Pelvic Lift   *Fig. 24   p. 127*

⑤ Medium Head Lift   *Fig. 25   p. 132*

⑥ Arm Rotations   *Fig. 30   p. 151*

⑦ Low to Medium Chin Lift   *Fig. 26   p. 136*

⑧ Medium Pelvic Lift   *Fig. 24   p. 127*

⑨ Medium Head Lift   *Fig. 25   p. 132*

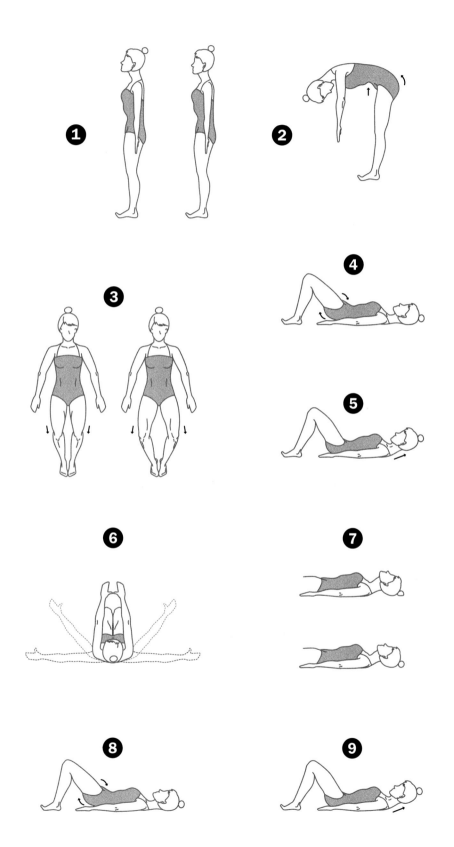

PLAN 4

(1) Foot Movements   *Fig. 18   p. 104*

(2) Medium Pelvic Lift   *Fig. 24   p. 127*

(3) Medium Head Lift   *Fig. 25   p. 132*

(4) Leg Rotations   *Fig. 20   p. 112*

(5) Low to Medium Chin Lift   *Fig. 26   p. 136*

(6) Narrow to Medium Knee Spreads   *Fig. 22   p. 122*

(7) Pelvic Bridge   *Fig. 24   p. 127*

(8) Medium Head Lift   *Fig. 25   p. 132*

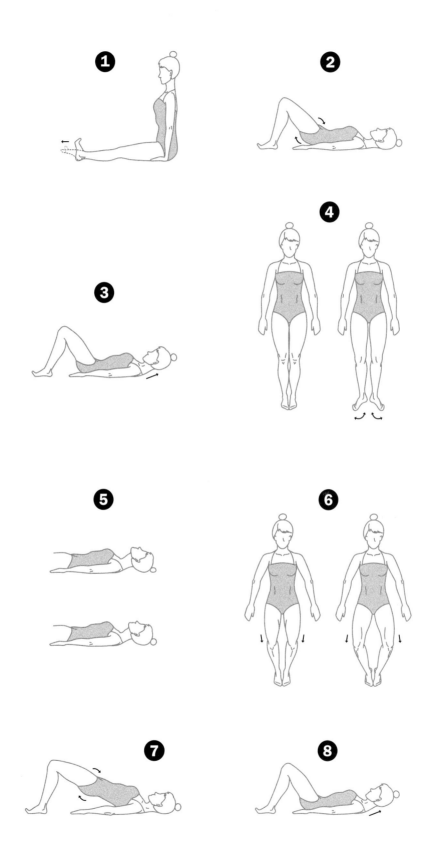

193

PLAN 5

① Hip Lift   *Fig. 21   p. 119*

② Leg Rotations   *Fig. 20   p. 112*

③ Medium Pelvic Lift   *Fig. 24   p. 127*

④ Medium Head Lift   *Fig. 25   p. 132*

⑤ Quarter Circle Arm Movements   *Fig. 31   p. 157*

⑥ Low to Medium Chin Lift   *Fig. 26   p. 136*

⑦ Medium Knee Spreads   *Fig. 22   p. 122*

⑧ Pelvic Bridge   *Fig. 24   p. 127*

⑨ Medium to Low Head Lift   *Fig. 25   p. 132*

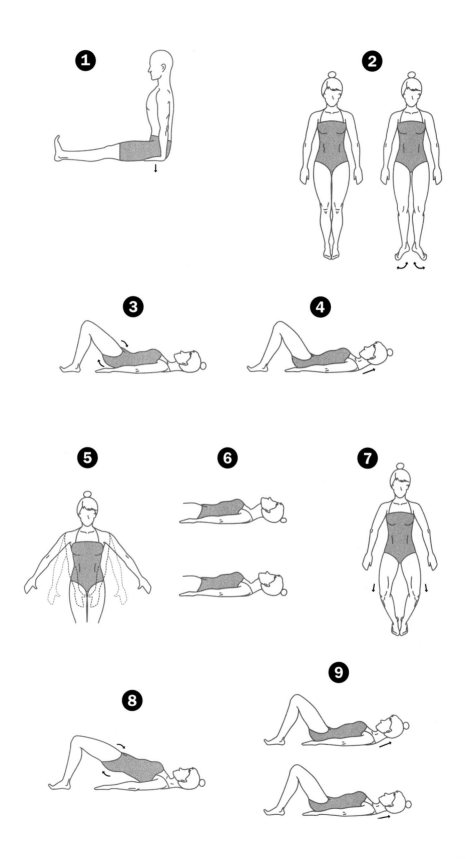

PLAN 6

① Knee Bends   *Fig. 39   p. 181*

② Leg Spreads   *Fig. 23   p. 125*

③ Shoulder Movements   *Fig. 29   p. 146*

④ Quarter Circle Arm Movements   *Fig. 31   p. 157*

⑤ Whole Circle Arm Movements   *Fig. 33   p. 161*

⑥ Chin Lifts   *Fig. 26   p. 136*

⑦ Medium Pelvic Lift   *Fig. 24   p. 127*

⑧ Medium Head Lift   *Fig. 25   p. 132*

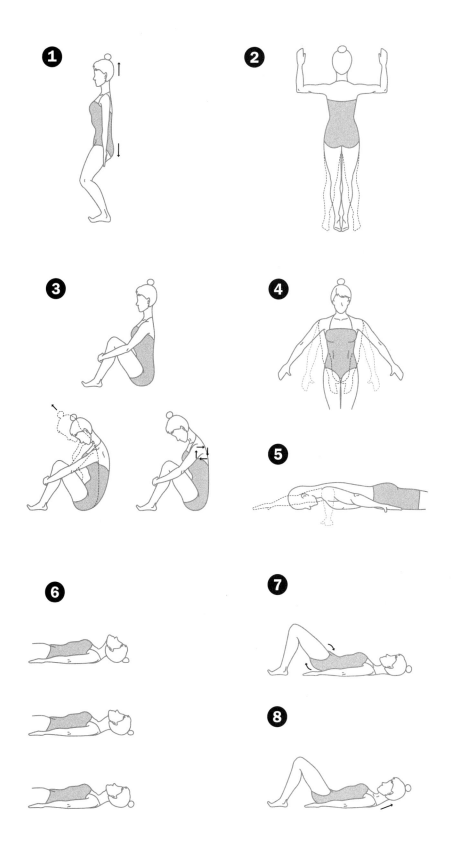

PLAN 7

①   **Sitting Erect**   *Fig. 37   p. 174*

②   **Rotational Movements of the Head**   *Fig. 37   p. 174*

③   **Rotational Movements of the Spine & Head**   *p. 176*

④   **Round Bends Sitting**   *Fig. 35   p. 167*

⑤   **Lateral Bends of the Head**   *Fig. 38   p. 179*

⑥   **Lateral Bends of the Trunk & Head**   *Fig. 38   p. 179*

⑦   **Forward Bends Sitting**   *Fig. 35   p. 167*

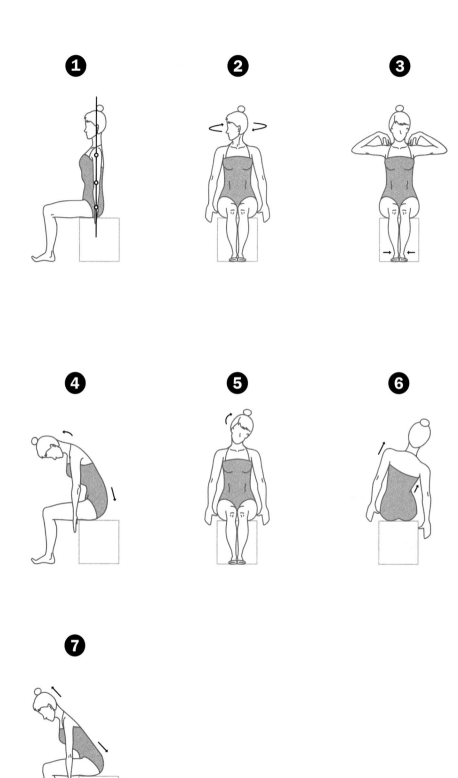

PLAN 8

① Forward Bends   *Fig. 35   p. 167–68*

② Medium Pelvic Lift   *Fig. 24   p. 127*

③ Low Head Lift   *Fig. 25   p. 132*

④ Reversal at Waistline   *Fig. 27   p. 138*

⑤ High Chin Lift   *Fig. 26   p. 136*

⑥ Medium Pelvic Lift   *Fig. 24   p. 127*

⑦ Reversal between Shoulders   *Fig. 27   p. 138*

⑧ Medium Pelvic Lift   *Fig. 24   p. 127*

⑨ Low Head Lift   *Fig. 25   p. 132*

⑩ Medium Knee Spreads to Sprawls   *Fig. 22   p. 122*

⑪ Cat Positions   *Fig. 28   p. 143*

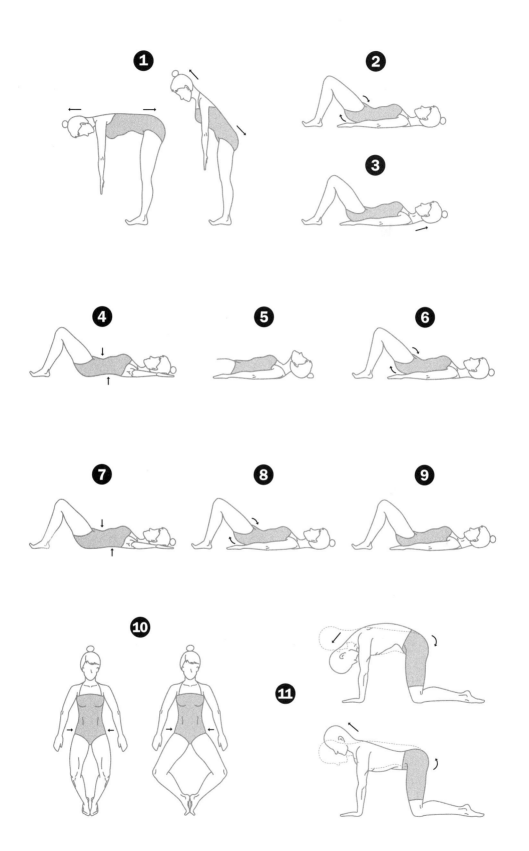

A PARTING WORD

My intention in writing this book was to provide information and corrective movements to those who want to help themselves maintain a good and healthy life. Knowledge of the probable cause of illness and pain will allow them to take action for preventative healing.

Every day, about 75 percent of the people I see, young and old, are walking or standing in an unhealthy manner that will eventually cause a health issue. Their lack of knowledge of natural, balanced body alignment and movement, along with a lack of awareness of their own body habits of walking and standing, will eventually get their attention from pain or illness.

Even though holistic and medical treatments may ease their discomfort, they will only be a temporary fix. Unless people retrain their neuromuscular systems to move in a natural, balanced form, all areas and systems of their bodies will continue to have negative effects.

My goal is to empower people with knowledge and understanding of the body's systems and body alignment. The movements of Dailey Inner Core Workout, based on a method created by a medical doctor with osteopathic training, have benefited so many of my students in amazing ways; I wanted to provide the masses with a successful self-help plan that can be applicable to each reader's daily life.

REFERENCES

Barry, Patricia. "The Side Effects of Side Effects." *AARP Bulletin*, September 2011, 14-16.

Bortz II, Walter. 1996. *Dare to Be 100*. New York: Fireside.

Castrone, Linda. "The Shape of Things to Come." *Rocky Mountain News*, March 6, 1995.

Darwin, Charles. 1872. *The Expression of the Emotions in Man and Animals*. London: John Murray.

Doi, Emi, and Michael Zielenziger. "Want to live to be 100? Try the Okinawa lifestyle." *Dallas Morning News*, December 14, 2001.

Ellis, John M. "Response of vitamin B-6 deficiency and the carpal tunnel syndrome to pyridoxine." *Proceedings of the National Academy of Science of the United States of America* 79 (December 1982): 7494-98.

Feldenkrais, Moshe. 1950. *Body and Mature Behavior*. New York: International Universities Press.

Feldman, Megan. "Put Me In Coach." *Dallas Observer*, September 24, 2009.

Fletcher, Ron A. 1978. *Every Body Is Beautiful*. Philadelphia: J. B. Lippincott.

Hagan, R. Donald, Babs R. Soller, Ye Yang, Stuart M. C. Lee, Cassie Wilson. "Noninvasive determination of exercise-induced hydrogen ion threshold through direct optical measurement." *Journal of Applied Physiology* 104, no. 3 (March 1, 2008): 837-44.

Hall, Stephen S. "A molecular code links emotions, mind and health," *Smithsonian*, June 1989, 62-71.

Hay, Louise L. 1988. *Heal Your Body, The Mental Causes of Physical Illness and the Metaphysical Way to Overcome Them.* Carson, CA: Hay House.

Kendall, Florence Peterson, Elizabeth Kendall McCreary, Patricia Geise Provance, Mary McIntyre Rodgers, and William Anthony Romani. 2005. *Muscles Testing and Function with Posture and Pain.* 5th ed. Baltimore: Lippincott Williams & Wilkins.

Lad, Vasant. 1985. *Ayurveda The Science of Self-Healing.* 2nd ed. Wilmot, WI: Lotus Press.

Lamb, David R. 1978. *Physiology of Exercise.* New York: *Macmillan.*

Listful, Emily. "Stay Healthy, Meditation 101." *Parade Magazine, Dallas Morning News,* January 23, 2011.

Menaker, Drusilla. "How to Live to Be 100: Secrets to a long life offered by Azerbaijan." *Dallas Morning News,* April 6, 2001.

Moritz, Andreas. 2009. *Cancer Is Not a Disease—It's a Survival Mechanism.* 3rd ed. Breingsville, PA: Ener-chi Wellness Press.

——. 2007. *The Amazing Liver & Gallbladder Flush.* 5th ed. Breingsville, PA: Ener-chi Wellness Press.

Moritz-Naisbitt, John. 1982. *Megatrends.* New York: Warner Books.

Ornish, Dean. 1992. *Dr. Dean Ornish's Program for Reversing Heart Disease.* New York: Ballantine Books.

Orr, Ken. "Reflexology: Ancient Healing Art & 21st Century Science," http://www.MassagingDallas.com.

Parker, Randall. "Facial Bone Aging Contributes to Aged Appearances." October 10, 2006. http://www.futurepundit.com/archives/003800.html.

Prakash, Om. 2012. *From Change to Transformation & Beyond.* Blooming, IN: iUniverse.

Schopenhauer, Arthur. "The World as Will and Representation," http://www.p2pilatesplus.com.

Sheldon, William Herbert. 1954. *Atlas of Men.* New York: Gramercy.

Smity, Eileen Keavy. 2000. *The Quick & Easy Ayurvedic Cookbook.* North Clarendon, VT: Tuttle.

Whitney, Craig R. "World's oldest known person dies at age 122." *New York Times*, August 5, 1997.

ACKNOWLEDGMENTS

Grateful appreciation goes to: Betty Black for asking me in 1980 to join her in teaching aerobic dance classes, which launched my exercise career; Nan Pipe Moore and her mother, who introduced me to a friend who taught aerobic dance classes in California and had taken a workshop with Ron Fletcher, author of *Every Body Is Beautiful* and a first-generation Pilates instructor in California; a buyer for Neiman Marcus Mail Order, who brought me the address of Ron Fletcher, whose studio phone number was unlisted due to the many movie stars who attended his classes and private instruction.

In my pioneering efforts to bring the Pilates method to Dallas, my appreciation extends to: Barbara Jean Coffman, a role model for the benefits she achieved from Ron Fletcher at his Hollywood studio, which her home town family and friends noticed; Glenda Nave, Mary Noel Lamont, Sally Bonnette, and Barbara Thomas Lemon for helping me put together Ron's first workshop in Dallas in May 1981; Larry Lane for recommending a studio for me to teach the first Pilates Mat classes in Dallas; Elise Murchison for her encouraging belief in the growth of my classes; Hara Hunt and Kay Tinsley, who provided space for me to teach Pilates Reformer lessons.

Appreciation for assisting me on my life journey as a fitness educator and the influence of the fine arts in my life, beginning during my formative years in Durant, OK, goes to my teachers: James Frazier, dance; Mrs. W. A. Lemon, piano; Ron Fletcher, who introduced me to the original Pilates Contrology of Joe and Clara Pilates, Ron's combination of the Pilates and Martha Graham approaches to movement, and Ron's advice that I pursue a degree in Exercise Physiology because people would listen only to women with a degree; osteopathic doctors Neil Pruzzo and Conrad Speece;

nutritionist Dr. Ron Overberg; Physio-Synthesis teachers Dr. Lucille Cochran, Roberta Reinecke, and Ida Thomas; Adriana Hardy and Tracy Roybal, who teach Feldenkraise Awareness through Movement; Ilana Pomeranz, who teaches Alexander Technique; Professor Allen Jackson, PhD, who advised me and calculated the statistics on my master's degree thesis.

My daughter Megan Dailey, illustrator and graphic designer for this book, and my husband, John Dailey, my computer and writing guide; Janica Smith; Julia Chester; editor Lauren Hidden; and the lessons I learned from many students who overcame physical problems through their regular participation in the Dailey Inner Core Workout.

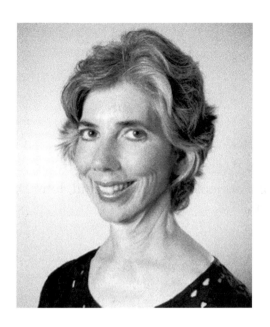

ABOUT THE AUTHOR

Alice Ann Dailey, MS, began her career as an elementary school classroom music and piano teacher. Her teaching career transitioned into physical fitness, and she became the first Pilates teacher in Dallas, Texas. She owned an exercise studio, Oasis Mind-Body Conditioning Center, and later taught PE Pilates at Booker T. Washington High School for the Performing and Visual Arts.

Dailey's education includes a bachelor of music degree in piano performance from the University of Oklahoma and a master of science degree in exercise physiology from the University of North Texas, which included an internship at the Sports Medicine Clinic of North Texas in Dallas. Her master's thesis, "The Relationship of the Sit and Reach Test to Criterion Measures of Hamstring and Back Flexibility in Young Females," was published in *Research Quarterly for Exercise and Sport* 57 (3) in September 1986, with Allen W. Jackson and Alice Ann Baker. She earned an American College of Sports Medicine Fitness Instructor Certification in 1985 and the Pilates Method Alliance Gold Certified Instructor in 2005.

The author's honors include: Marquis Who's Who in Medicine and Health Care, 1997; IDEA Master Level Personal Fitness Trainer, 2000; Marquis Who's Who in Education, 2003; International Educator of Year—International Biographical Center of Cambridge, England, 2004; International Biographical Center's Leading Educators of the World, 2005. In 2001, she hosted with Ellen Locy a thirteen-and-a-half-hour fitness series, "Your Dailey Inner Body Workout."

Her mission in writing *Dailey Strengthening: 6 Keys to Balance Core Muscles for Optimal Health* is to provide the information she has learned from her students and her own self-healing experiences so that others may create a plan to maintain their body, mind, and spirit in good health.

INDEX OF ILLUSTRATIONS

Fig. 1	damaged & dead hearing cells	20
Fig. 2	ideal alignment: posterior view	32
Fig. 3	faulty alignment: lateral tilt	33
Fig. 4	ideal alignment: side view	35
Fig. 5	faulty alignment: posterior tilt	36
Fig. 6	faulty alignment: anterior tilt	37
Fig. 7	respiratory system	41
Fig. 8	respiration	42
Fig. 9	skeletal muscle: structural layers of muscle to muscle fibers	55
Fig. 10	inner ear balance sensors	61
Fig. 11	vertical line posture	75
Fig. 12	six structural triangles	80–81
Fig. 13	balanced & unbalanced knees	82
Fig. 14	foot alignment	82
Fig. 15	sitting: legs extended & supine	84
Fig. 16	cranial motion on inhalation & exhalation	86
Fig. 17	occipital pump on inhalation & exhalation	88
Fig. 18	foot movements	104
Fig. 19	forward heel raises	110
Fig. 20	leg rotations	112
Fig. 21	hip lift	119
Fig. 22	knee spreads	122
Fig. 23	leg spreads	125
Fig. 24	pelvic tilts & lifts	127
Fig. 25	head lifts	132
Fig. 26	chin lifts	136
Fig. 27	reversals	138
Fig. 28	cat positions	143
Fig. 29	shoulder movements	146
Fig. 30	arm rotations	151
Fig. 31	quarter circle arm movements	157
Fig. 32	half circle arm movements	159

Fig. 33	whole circle arm movements	161
Fig. 34	forward & backward sways	165
Fig. 35	forward bends	167–68
Fig. 36	forward bends: kneeling	172–73
Fig. 37	rotational movements	174
Fig. 38	lateral bends	179
Fig. 39	knee bends	181